Remembering the Music, Forgetting the Words

Travels with Mom in the Land of Dementia

Kate Whouley

Beacon Press, Boston

Beacon Press
25 Beacon Street
Boston, Massachusetts 02108-2892
www.beacon.org

Beacon Press books
are published under the auspices of
the Unitarian Universalist Association of Congregations.

14 13 12 11   8 7 6 5 4 3 2 1

This book is printed on acid-free paper that meets the uncoated paper
ANSI/NISO specifications for permanence as revised in 1992.

Text design and composition by Wilsted & Taylor Publishing Services

The individuals mentioned in this narrative
are actual persons. In a few cases, names or identifying traits
have been changed or blurred for reasons of privacy.

Library of Congress Cataloging-in-Publication Data
Whouley, Kate.
Remembering the music, forgetting the words :
travels with Mom in the land of dementia / Kate Whouley.
p. cm.
ISBN 978-0-8070-0319-0 (hardcover : acid-free paper)
1. Whouley, Kate. 2. Whouley, Kate—Family. 3. Alzheimer's
disease—Patients—United States—Family relationships.
4. Alzheimer's disease—Patients—United States—Biography.
5. Mothers and daughters—United States. I. Title.
RC523.2.W495 2011
616.8'31—dc22   2011012351

For Jack

Contents

Chapter One

What We Don't Know

I don't know my mother has Alzheimer's.

What I don't know, what she will never know—soon it will be killing both of us. But not quite yet. On this particular day, we are in the time and space that, soon enough, I will think of as *before*. We are unknowing—my mother and I—and we are happy.

Today—a late May Saturday in 2004—my first book will be launched with a party at a venerable Cape Cod bookstore. You can find Titcomb's Bookshop by looking for the man out front in the tricornered hat. Ted, son of Ralph and Nancy Titcomb, made the man in art school and placed him in his parents' front yard, which also happens to be the front yard of the bookstore. Positioned near the bookstore sign, the wrought-iron gentle-man carrying a walking stick—and, of course, a book—has become something of a landmark on scenic Route 6A. I'm not sure anyone knows who he is supposed to be. Ben Franklin? Daniel Webster? Does his red coat suggest he is British? Nor do many folks know why he's there. But if you suggest meeting at the bookstore with the statue of that colonial guy out front, pretty much everybody who lives here—book reader or not—knows just where that is.

Before the party begins, you'll find me in and out of the

Titcombs' kitchen. I am accompanied by my stepsister, Vicki, and her partner, Martha. We are delivering beer and May wine, platters of fruit and cheese, toothpicks with miniature whirligigs attached to one end, boxes of crackers, bags of ice, paper plates, napkins, and a giant sheet cake frosted with an image of the book jacket. We're expecting 85 guests, based on the RSVPs to the 131 invitations I sent out about a month ago.

In a red silk V-neck and a voluminous black parachute skirt—both unfortunate choices for the photos my friend Anne will insist on taking—I am not dressed like a bride, but the planning and execution of this event has felt a lot like managing a wedding. I swear that's why my uncle Jack offered to pay for hotel rooms for family members who wanted to come to the party. He'd done the same a year earlier, when my cousin (his nephew) Josh married Cindy in a breathtaking setting way the hell up in the mountains of Vermont. I am now forty-five years old, unmarried, and without a date for my own party. Jack, I am pretty sure, has deduced he is unlikely to walk me down the aisle. In lieu of giving away the aging bride, he would make it possible for far-flung family to come to my book party.

Vicki and Martha arrived late Thursday, driving seven hours from Bangor, Maine. On Friday they ran errands, picked up food and beverages, and figured out how to fit everything into my already overloaded refrigerator. They were the perfect bridesmaids. The maid of honor for my Book Wedding is my dear friend, Tina. She arrived Friday night in time to nurse me through my predictable wardrobe crisis. After deciding the black palazzo pants and lacy zip-up top I'd planned to wear would be too hot and too dressy, I splurged on an alternative outfit at a Hyannis boutique—the kind of place where the owner can convince you that you look amazing, and some of the time, you do.

"Does this shirt make me look completely top-heavy?"

Tina, stretched out on my bed, told me that I had a great top, that I should be proud of it. My friend and I nurture a mutual admiration of our differences. She wishes for a fuller bust; I wish for her neat figure. I wish for curls in my hair, while she wishes for the straightness of mine. Our friendship runs much deeper, but the mutual admiration of our inverses makes both of us feel better.

∽

The planning and attendants may suggest "alternative wedding," but in terms of momentous, life-changing events, this party celebrates my best entry yet in the category of child substitutes.

"If you don't give me grandchildren," my mother once said to me, "give me books." I was in my mid-twenties at the time and, I believed, more apt to have children than to birth books. It seemed to me a weird thing to say—and premature. I was just out of a six-year off-again, on-again relationship with my college sweetheart, but I didn't consider myself ineligible for a future relationship—or a family.

"Huh?" I managed.

"Not everyone has children these days. Though it would be nice if you found someone and got married. I'd *like* grandchildren. But if you wrote a book or two instead, that would be okay with me."

My mother's willingness to embrace literary progeny was no doubt rooted in her working life: she was first a high school English teacher and later the coordinator of English for her school system. It was a job she was born to do and a job she very nearly didn't get. We had moved just the year before, and she was new to the department. She was younger than the other

candidates and the first woman to apply for a coordinator position in the system.

My mother knew she wouldn't win a popularity contest
with her colleagues—men or women—by refusing to accept
the status quo. But she believed she was qualified, deserving of
consideration, and only coincidentally female. When she was
not invited for an interview, she did not accept her fate. She
wrote letters, made phone calls, and asked for a meeting with
superintendent. Finally she was told she could appear before the
school committee to be interviewed—at midnight on a school
night.

Picture it: a midnight interview, grudgingly granted, with
every person in the room viewing you as nothing more than a
loudmouthed thorn in his side, resenting your persistence, your
very presence in the room, not to mention your sex. And it's
been, after all, a long night, and goddamn it, can't we just get
this coordinator thing over with? Enter my mother: striking,
young, with a trained voice that projects from her diaphragm
as she makes a killer presentation, outlines a bold new direction
for the English department, a direction that will position the
school system as an educational leader, a direction that will lead
to commendations and awards and grant money.

Sometime in the wee hours of the morning the vote was
taken, and my mother was the new coordinator of English.

I was not yet twelve years old when my mother got that job,
but the way she fought for it—and won—is absolutely tangled
up in who I am today. She was my heroine in those days—we
were on our own, and she was an accidental feminist icon. I was
proud of my mom, proud of her job, and proud of her polyester
pantsuits.

Today, the Welcome Day for her first grandbook, my
mother is subdued. She's leaning on Bill's elbow, smiling and

making polite conversation as folks approach her. She makes no effort to circulate. I know that her arthritic hip is probably bothering her. But that's not the whole story. My mom hasn't been herself since the cancer—breast cancer. Surgery, radiation—no chemo, because she has a chronic kidney condition. They found it early—stage one—and almost two years have passed since she finished her treatment. She is cancer free. But it isn't just the cancer that is gone. Some of the grit that got her that job, some of the spark and the mischief that won over her reluctant colleagues—hell, even some of the sarcasm I have not always appreciated—have departed with those poisoned cells. As I watch her from across the room, I have this unshakable sense that my *real* mother is not here.

Pushing that thought aside, I position myself in the far corner of the bookstore, at the book-signing table that has been set up for me. In my life as a bookseller, I hosted many authors, passing the books, open to the title page, to such literary luminaries as Doris Lessing, Mario Vargas Llosa, and Andre Dubus. Once, I provided Powdermilk biscuits for Garrison Keillor. Sitting behind the author desk today feels exciting, and also odd. But at least I know what to do.

Four years ago yesterday, I moved a tiny two-room cottage and positioned it next to my three-room home on Cape Cod. Over the span of the next nine months, the two cottages were, as my builder liked to say, "married together." The story of the move—and the marriage—formed the basis for the book that is now stacked beside me on the table: *Cottage for Sale, Must Be Moved.*

A steady stream of folks visit me at my corner station, many of them wearing the pins that identify anyone who is mentioned in the book. I'd ordered custom buttons from an irresistibly named Internet presence called the Button King, but they didn't arrive in time for the party. I made do, inserting miniature images of the book cover photo into clear badge holders I'd found at Staples. My creations require some Scotch tape to hold the vertical images in place, and the badges have to be worn sideways, but they still work their magic: lending courage to otherwise reserved New Englanders. "Who are you in the book?" It's the perfect conversation starter.

As folks hand over their books to be signed, I discover that I am not the only person signing books at this party. There are almost as many signatures as there are entries in the Cast and Crew list at the front of the book. I see that the house mover, Mr. Hayden, has signed next to his name; my father-and-son building team, Ed and John, have signed their names too. I see my mother's signature, and Tina's; my friends Harry and Tony, a.k.a. the Bog Boys, have signed books. The makeshift badges have presented not only an easy introduction, but also an opportunity for autographs. I am thrilled by this unexpected development, and I notice all of the other people signing books look pretty happy too.

My friend Anne, with her radio and television voice, takes the microphone that Harry, a musician, has provided, along with a portable amp. "Isn't she the woman from Channel Two?" several folks have already asked me while I was signing their books. That's WGBH, the Boston public television affiliate, where Anne's smiling face and lovely manner work together to coax dollars from viewers several times a year. Anne is just as effective behind the camera. She can talk even the most camera-shy individual into posing for her—and even better, she helps the photophobic relax, making for great pictures every time.

Before I read, Anne uses the mike to organize folks so they will be able to hear. Some folks she settles on the stairs; she makes certain anyone who needs a seat—like my mother—has one. I realize the work she is doing now isn't unlike the way she must organize those giant group shots she takes at weddings, though in this case she is placing people so I can be heard rather than so they can be seen.

I read. I've selected a series of short bits that showcase some of the most important partygoers: Mr. Hayden, Ed, John, the Bog Boys. While I am reading, you can hear the proverbial pin drop in the space. I realize I have their attention and that, at some point, every single person in the space is caught up in the story. I take this as a good sign.

After the reading, John comes over to say hello. "The girls were disappointed when you stopped. They asked if I could read the rest of the story to them when we get home." I take it as a huge compliment that Katelin and Nicole—ages six and eight, dolled up in party dresses and twirling around their father— were engaged in the story.

"You guys don't have badges on, and you're in the book— would you like a pin like your dad's?"

"Yes!"

"Yes!"

As I pin little cottages onto their dresses, I realize there have already been so many special moments at this party that I'm not sure I could pick out one as my favorite.

But there is still one coming. One that will be perfect, and perfectly bittersweet. Anne will make that moment. She will round up my mother and lead her over to my corner, position her next to me, and ask us to look up and smile. And we will. Because we are still operating in that time and space that will become *before*. We are okay. Happy; maybe even a little high. The party is buzzing. There is laughter and goodwill all around us. It is a celebration: I've brought my mother's first grandbook into the world. And what we don't know—it isn't killing us yet.

Chapter Two

Eating Cake

In second grade, I wrote this for a school assignment: "My mother is a drama couch. She has dark brown hair, big blue eyes and is very pretty." By way of illustration, I'd drawn a picture of my mother with the aforementioned dark brown hair and big blue eyes, set off nicely by a blue turtleneck. About my father, I composed a rhyme: "My father's name is Paul, and he is very tall. My father's hair is black, and handsomeness he does not lack." My father, drawn with brown eyes and black hair, was extra skinny, with the suggestion of height—he was six-five. I also wrote two sentences about my cat, Timothy, in this same assignment, but I don't remember the words, only the picture, which was of an all-black cat standing, tail up, next to a red food bowl.

"C-o-*a*-c-h: coach." My mother corrected me when I brought the papers home to show her. "You spelled it like I was the living room couch, c-o-*u*-c-h." It was an important distinction, because although my classroom teacher had corrected the spelling, she had not explained that I had confused my lovely and exciting mother with a piece of overstuffed furniture. "I like the turtleneck," my mother added. My father, on the other hand, had no quarrels with my spelling or my assessment. "And handsomeness I do not lack," he took to repeating for several months after I completed the assignment.

When I think about what I chose to write about each of my parents—and this back in the middle sixties—I am struck that I led with my mother's work life and didn't mention my father's work at all. Having a working mother was unusual in those days, but I don't think that's the only reason I brought it up in my assignment. My father, in my early childhood, held a succession of jobs that were mysterious to me. My mother's work I understood: she taught school and directed plays. I suspect, too, that by the time I was in second grade, I already knew something about my mother that would be true for many years to come: she was better at work than she was at home.

My mom, the drama coach, was known and respected throughout our community. The Cumberland High School Thespian Society, as they called themselves, were a consistent and formidable team in the regional, state, and (at least once) national one-act play competitions. My mother liked to brag that the drama kids brought home more trophies than the football team. She was willing to point this out to her principal and members of the school committee as required in order to get the funding she needed for her Thespians.

My favorite photograph of my mother was taken to accompany an article about the drama kids and their winning record. She is seated in the high school auditorium. You can see the empty seats around her. She is in profile, her head lifted up, her chin strong. She has on a white mock turtleneck, and the top of the neck has dainty scallops. Her long legs are crossed in the air, resting on the back of the seat in front of her, and you can see a stretch of calf and ankle beyond the capri-length jeans she's wearing. She has on little white Keds. On her left hand, her engagement ring is visible even as she gestures, her left palm up in the air. Around that wrist you see a charm bracelet, filled with the dangling filigree charms the kids gave her after each production. Also a watch. You can tell she is either about to say something or has just said it—something like *Wait* or *Take your time with that line* or *Move more slowly on that entrance.*

My mother was a beautiful woman, and in this picture with her short dark hair, her perfectly arched brow, and her youthful good looks, she is a vision of glamour and authority. I love the photo not only because it shows my mother in her full glory but because it reminds me of a time in our life together, a time that I loved. I was never more content than I was tagging along to my mother's rehearsals. I was in awe of the high school kids, and I loved watching the stories acted out on stage. I was struck by how the kids offstage did or didn't match up with their characters, and intrigued to see the same kids take entirely different roles from one production to the next. And I loved hearing my mother calling out from the darkness of the auditorium: "I'm losing that line. Project from your diaphragm!"

The productions I remember best were a bouquet of light and dark: *The Wizard of Oz*, *Finian's Rainbow*, *One with the Flame*, and *Murder in the Cathedral*. The first two were well-known musicals, the latter two one-act plays—one about Joan of Arc, the other about the Archbishop of Canterbury. I'm not sure, upon reflection, whether my mother's choice in one-acts had anything to do with her Catholic school education or whether—more likely—she was drawn to the power of those plays and knew she had just the right Thespian to play the doomed and dramatic lead in each. An important consideration, if the drama kids were to keep bringing home the trophies.

I don't recall ever being bored at those evening rehearsals. If the action on stage became repetitive, I'd troll the auditorium for lost pencils and the occasional coin dropped by the kids who came to the auditorium by day for study hall. I'd puzzle over the odd bit of tiny graffiti carved into the underside of one of the wooden armrests between the seats. I'd move around the auditorium like a secret agent, trying out different seats to check out the views.

My mother, sometimes working with kids who could act but not sing, or kids who looked the part but had trouble acting it, came up with creative ways to achieve the required effect. I remember her rearranging more than one song into what we'd now think of as rap versions, asking her kids to speak it in rhythm rather than sing it. Those moments of artistic breakthrough were my favorite. My mother would move close to the stage, gather all the kids around, and explain what she had in mind. She'd read the lines herself, demonstrate. I would stand close to her, taking her in, proud of her, proud of the way all the kids hung on her every move, her every word. She'd ask them to try it and try again. She'd make small corrections, murmur encouragement, adjust their positioning on stage. Then she would move back, deeper into the auditorium, resume her position. And inhabit the photograph that now sits in a small frame on my living room mantel.

The photograph captures another *before* moment: it was a time before my father left the family, before my parents divorced, before my mother met and married her second husband, before her life—and mine—changed in ways that would have uncontrollable consequences. In this moment, my mother is directing, and the kids on the stage will do exactly what she says.

‿

It's the day after the book party. All I want to do is sleep, but duty—and a concert—calls. I play flute in the Cape Cod

Conservatory Concert Band, and this is the last concert of our season.

"We had fun yesterday," John says when he sees me backstage. In a rare crossover of my musical life with the rest of my life, I'd invited three people from the band to the book launch: Tom, the tuba player, who as the head of the health department has a cameo appearance in the book; Susan, who sits next to me in the flute section; and the band's director, John, who came with his wife, Darlene.

"Thanks for coming." I am not sure what else to say. I've played flute under John's baton for ten years now, sitting just a few feet from his left elbow. I've joked with him that I wouldn't know how to follow if I were seated straight on—I'm so used to watching his movements in profile. John depends on me to play the part, to keep my wits about me during the tough spots and the solos. I depend on him to keep the beat and to throw me an extra large cue when he senses that I need it. It's a strange sort of closeness, a musical intimacy fueled with mutual respect. Yet we have no particular relationship outside the band. That's true for many of my musical colleagues in the ensemble. We show up; we play. We go home.

For me, the interesting part about the band is that we show up. Every year, starting in late September and ending in late May, we gather on Monday nights to rehearse. Because our practice space is in an elementary school, we don't rehearse on Monday holidays or during school vacation weeks. For this reason, band feels a little like being back in school, and when school lets out for the summer, there is a part of me that revels in my Monday night freedom—which begins tomorrow night.

On stage today, we will number fifty musicians. We are the wind and percussion equivalent of a "pops" orchestra. Our programs blend classical selections, Broadway numbers, film music, tunes from the American songbook, some contemporary music—including a couple of premieres—and of course the requisite march. Among our members are two semiretired doctors, one an allergist, the other a psychiatrist; several teachers, active and retired; an investment banker; a surgical nurse; a town administrator; a yoga instructor; a retired reverend; and a high school music director. Some of us play beautifully and some play well; some just okay. Some of us stumble through our parts when we read through the music for our next concert. Some of us sight-read like pros. Some of us are pros, if we are to define professional the way they used to in the Olympics. Are we ever paid to play? Yes. Some of us are paid to play. But not at this gig. Today, and every Monday night, we are playing for free. Or if you want to be absolutely accurate: we are paying to play.

At the beginning of each school year, when the band reassembles after a summer off, we pay our dues. It was ten dollars for a long time, then the amount doubled to twenty. There were some grumbles about that until we came to understand that only half of it would go to the conservatory from whom we borrow the music library; the other half would go to buy us new music. This year we were asked for forty dollars. John, appalled at the conservatory demands, was apologetic. But most of us just sighed and forked over the cash.

Demographically, band membership skews white and over sixty. It isn't that we don't welcome younger players or that we are exclusionary in any way. The demographics of Cape Cod skew pretty much the same way. And then there is the music we play. It's band music. If it didn't seem cool in high school, it isn't likely to grow on you. That lack of cool sometimes makes it tough to get an audience. And yet, contrary to what you might imagine, these fifty or so aging band geeks make good music together. When the local papers give us some coverage, we'll draw an audience of a hundred and fifty or two hundred people who will tap, clap, and cheer. They will leave the auditorium humming and happy.

Today my mom and Bill are in the audience. "He's not my boyfriend," she insisted when I teased her about the man she had met through some volunteer work a few years ago.

"Gentleman friend," I suggested.

"Friend," she said. "I'm too old for all that other stuff. And he's older than me."

My mom is sixty-eight. Bill is somewhere in his mid-seventies, a semi-retired engineer who, as best as I can figure, seems to be working pretty much full-time. I like him. My mother's siblings like him. My mother likes him. And best of all, he likes my mother. Bill lost his wife to cancer a few years before he met my mother. I am not certain that he feels like he is "too old for all that other stuff."

"Companion," I suggested, because it seems to me that Bill accompanies my mother most places—yesterday to the party, today to the concert—and I know they eat dinner and watch a movie at his place every Friday night.

"Companion," my mother repeated. "Okay. Yes, I like that."

After the concert, my mother and her companion come back to my house, where I serve them party leftovers. For dessert, there is the book jacket cake.

"Busy weekend. You must be exhausted, Katie," my mother says. Bill nods.

I've changed out of my concert formalwear and into jeans. Really, I don't feel the exhaustion yet, because I am always wired after I play a concert. But I know it is there. "I will be a zombie tomorrow," I say. "But I might stay high all night if I keep eating cake."

"This cake . . ." my mother says. "It is *sooo* good!"

"Isn't it?" From my deck, we watch the sun drop behind the treetops. My mother excuses herself and moves to the front garden. A bench there is designated as the smoking lounge. When she returns from her cigarette break, we achieve instant and unanimous agreement on seconds. Content, blissful, ensconced in the safety of *before*, we eat another slice of chocolate cake.

Chapter Three

Minding My Business

As spring turns to summer, I suspect that all is not well with Mom. She seems off to me—off in a way that no one else would notice. I've been blaming the cancer diagnosis, but we're two years past treatment and something is still not right. I think I need to spend more time with her. But instead, I find myself driving around New England on a low-budget book tour, checking in with my mother long-distance. She tells me funny stories about her cat, Emily—her second cat named Emily, after Emily Dickinson—and in the middle of one story that she has already told me, I wonder, *Does she remember she had another cat named Emily?*

I also wonder, when Christmas comes, why she declares she will not decorate this year. My mother, the Christmas Queen, the proud owner of an ever-growing Santa collection, not decorate?

"I can come over and help," I offer.

"No—no!" she says, with more emphasis than is required.

It occurs to me that whenever we do something together, she is already at her front door, waiting for me, when I pull into the driveway. I realize, with a horrible feeling in the pit of my stomach, that she is keeping me out of her house. Just like she did when she was drinking.

No. *Please. No.*

I've always hated the expression, "Be careful what you wish for."

In wishing, hoping, praying that my mother hasn't started drinking again, I am not making myself clear to God, or to the Intentional Universe, or to Whimsical Fate. I forget to say, *Also, please don't let it be dementia.*

∽

My mother and Bill are headed to New Hampshire for the weekend—he to his daughter's house, and my mother to visit my aunt Rosemary—and I am to feed Emily. After all these months of keeping me out of her house, my mother has asked me to cross her threshold.

Walking in, I am assaulted by the stench. The closeness of the air and the infusion of cigarette smoke in the very walls of the house do not mask the smell of rotting food that transports me in time to another house, to the same smell.

When my mother was hospitalized ten years ago—the hospitalization that led to the end of her drinking days—a cop showed up while we were in the emergency room. "This is her daughter," the nurse had said, leading him to me. I suggested we step out to the lobby, not wanting to conduct whatever surreal conversation we were about to have within earshot of my mother.

"My name is Kate," I told him, fearful my mother had been in an accident that I didn't know about. Thoughts raced through my head: *Driving drunk? Oh my God! What else could it be? Has someone been hurt?* I waited for him to speak.

"We got a call from one of the neighbors," he began. "They hadn't seen your mother for several days, but her car was there."

I nodded, not sure where this was going. "We knocked on the door, and there was no response. The slider was open, so we went in, to make sure she was okay, you know."

"Uh-huh."

"Well, I don't know if you've been in there—"

"She hasn't let me in her house in over a year."

"Well, ma'am, the place isn't fit for human habitation. I'm gonna have to report it to the board of health. Have it condemned."

"*Condemned?*" I remember that moment, standing in the lobby of Cape Cod Hospital, my mother back in the ER waiting to be admitted for dehydration, malnourishment, and who knew what else, and a cop—a cop!—telling me that her house would be condemned. I felt like I was in some extra awful made-for-TV movie.

"It's not fit for habitation," he repeated. "I have to report it."

"Well, can you give me a chance to take care of it? I mean— I've been here at the hospital with my mother. But I have every intention of going over there and cleaning up as soon as she's admitted."

"It's nothing you can clean yourself," he said, not unkindly.

"Well, I can get help. I can make arrangements. Please, can you give me a few days?" I wasn't sure what having your house condemned meant, really, but I was pretty sure it was an official status we had best avoid.

"Sure," he said after a pause. "I can give you a week, but I'll need to check back with you. My advice is you call one of those disaster-cleaning companies. The kind that cleans up after fires and such."

"I will. Right away. Thank you."

"Good luck," he said before he turned to leave the lobby.

I am grateful that cop isn't walking in behind me today.

The first thing you have to understand about my mother is that she likes stuff, and she likes her stuff on display. When she is well, my mother's home, while not to my taste, is decorated—arranged—with a sense of style. You can see there is a mind at work, a mind that has inventoried the stuff, has considered what will look best where, and has made sure that each object is in the place where it will be most visually pleasing.

One problem with her decorating style is it requires a hell of a lot of upkeep. It is clear to me, as I step inside the living room, that my mother has not been keeping up.

Is she drinking again? Could I have missed that?

I scan the floor: magazines, newspapers, open boxes of Christmas decorations, crumpled tissues, and the shiny gold bands from cigarette wrappers. No vodka bottles. I move into the kitchen, where the trail of coffee grounds reassures me she is restricting her liquid intake to her required eight cups a day.

The sink is filled with empty cat food cans; the counter, stacked with dirty dishes; the floor, littered with unopened mail.

The smell. Oh my God, the smell.

Keeping my mouth covered and my breathing shallow, I tour the rest of the house. In my mother's signature attempt to clean up, there are half-filled Hefty trash bags in every room. In her bedroom, all available surfaces, including the bed and the floor, are covered in clothing.

"I wanted to do some sorting for the Goodwill," she will tell me a few days later.

Where to begin?

I open every window, then I head for the kitchen. The cat food cans are beyond recycling. Some of the dishes are so encrusted with ancient, molding food that I toss them into one of the Hefty bags, whispering my apologies to the environment.

Staring at the cigarette butts floating in about five inches of brown water in the sink, I realize I need gloves.

Miracles are possible: I find an unopened pair of rubber gloves in the cabinet under the sink. An hour and a half later, I have claimed a beachhead: the sink and the countertop as far as the stove. I cannot bear to open the refrigerator.

I make a phone call.

The next day three cleaners arrive, and I work with them. Several hours later, we have made progress. I still have to figure out what to do with all the trash we have accumulated. For now, I stack the bags in the little breezeway off the kitchen.

"Thanks," my mother says to me when she returns from New Hampshire. "I'd been meaning to pick up, but I didn't have time before I went away for the weekend."

෴

Add extra turmeric to your sautés—but first throw out the anodized aluminum cookware. Forget the Puzzlemaster on NPR—it's not tough enough; start doing the *Times*'s Sunday crossword. Take up tai chi; learn to speak Mandarin. Eat fish while weightlifting.

It will be many months before well-meaning folks will give me tips about preventing Alzheimer's. Many months before I will want to scream at them, shake them, beg them to pay attention: *Do you realize what you are saying? I tell you my mother has Alzheimer's and you tell me how to prevent it? It's too late to prevent it! She has it!*

Do you think you're being subtle? I will want to ask them. *Of course I know I may be genetically predisposed to this terrible disease!* Yes, I've read about nutrition and toxicity and exercise and ways to keep my brain engaged. But the bottom line is: right now, in this moment, my awareness isn't important. This isn't about me. It's about my mother. She needs me. Way, way more than I need to take up Sudoku.

Not that she knows she needs me or would be willing to admit it if she did. In the early stages of Alzheimer's and related dementia, I will learn, the patient is often angered by your attempts to be helpful.

"It's none of your goddamn business, Kathleen!" my mother says, using my full given name and speaking in that warning voice that mothers acquire when their children enter the terrible twos. I am forty years away from toddlerhood, but I can feel my stomach muscles clench, the uncertainty set in. I am conditioned to link that voice with unpleasant, yet mostly untold, consequences. I back off—just as she knows I will.

After the great weekend cleanup, I am determined to maintain an acceptable level of cleanliness at my mother's house. I try a soft approach. We can all use help with cleaning, right? She is okay with my paying for her trash to be picked up every other week, but she doesn't want to let "a stranger" into her house to clean.

"Noelle is great," I assure her. "I've known her for years. She isn't a stranger. You'll like her." Variations on this conversation take place over the course of four more weeks. During those weeks I come to Mom's house, clean up the kitchen, do dishes, and talk about how it would be a lot easier on me if she would let Noelle do this for me. "And Noelle could use the work." I tell my mother how Noelle has her own business, has been cleaning houses since she was in her teens in order to help her own mother make ends meet.

At last she relents, but refuses to let Noelle into the bedroom—where the Goodwill sorting is an ongoing, never-ending, apparently top-secret job. In time, my mother begins to look forward to Noelle's biweekly visits. But she can't seem to learn her name. "I gave Michelle a check for ten dollars in a Christmas card," she tells me.

"Noelle," I say. "Not Michelle. Noelle. Like Christmas."

Unless I collect her for an outing, my mother sits, smoking, in the living room, making conversation as Noelle cleans around her. At least once, she persuades Noelle to just sit and chat. "Don't work so hard!" she tells her.

Noelle, reporting back to me, refuses to be paid for not cleaning, and I refuse her refusal. I pay Noelle, who is sanguine about my mother's propensity to rhyme her name rather than remember it and untroubled by her minimal tip. "Older people have a different idea about money," she explains to me.

I call my mother to remind her when the trash will be picked up and when Noelle is due for a visit. The arrangement isn't perfect: the house is not spotless; the trash men are sometimes locked out of the breezeway. But we have made progress, I tell myself. The truth of the matter is, like many family members who suspect something is wrong but are not yet sure what that something is, I want to believe my mother is okay—only in need of a little help around the house.

For now, we are satisfied. I have managed to create some order out of chaos. My mother, meanwhile, has created a diversion. While I am focused on keeping her house clean and tidy, she is safe from my deeper scrutiny.

When I mention the now neatly aligned but still-mounting pile of unopened mail on her coffee table, my mother says, "It's none of your goddamn business, Kathleen!"

If only our businesses could be so handily divided into hers and mine.

Chapter Four

House Hunt

Al is wearing a suit. A dark suit, with a crisp white shirt and a thin silk tie. I am wearing red: my knee-length holly-berry-red down parka. Together we look like a couple who forgot to do the wardrobe consult before we left home.

We're dressed, each in our way, for a day of house hunting.

"You know I'm just exploring options, right? I'm not in any position to act, even if we see something I like." We'd talked this through on the phone earlier in the week, but seeing Al in a suit makes me worry that he might be taking my explorations way too seriously. "I don't want to waste your time."

He smiles. "Kate, you are my first client ever. If you were a dollar bill, I'd paste you right here." He taps a space between the windshield visors. "I don't care if you buy anything. You're giving me a great chance to practice. And a way to see some of the inventory."

Inventory, meaning houses on the market. "Realtor talk. I'm impressed," I say teasingly. "But—you're sure this is okay?"

"Absolutely."

Eighteen years ago, when I was a twenty-eight-year-old homeowner in search of some help to manage my highly ir-regular lawn, a coworker named Betty told me her son had just started a landscaping business. When Al arrived to assess the situation, he was barely out of high school. He had a halo of golden curls and an unmistakable air of innocence. Though he lacked roundness of body, I swear he would have passed for a Sistine cherub if you just painted a little sky around his head. I found it hard to talk to him without blushing.

Over the past several years, Al has lost a good deal of his innocence to a messy divorce followed by rigorous and ongoing custody disagreements. If the years and the challenges of his life—and a shorter haircut—have eroded the angelic aspect of Al's countenance, they have also made him more handsome. Al has recently secured his real estate license. In his suit, he is impressive—gorgeous, to be precise. I'm used to seeing him in his landscaping greens, attached to a lawn mower or a Weedwacker and wearing ear protectors. Today I find myself sneaking glances at him while he drives us to our first appointment.

It's an antique colonial on Route 6A in Yarmouth Port. The listing agent who meets us in the driveway watches us climb out of the truck, then looks down at her notes before she approaches with an outstretched hand. This agent double take will occur at every stop on our house-hunting tour today. One agent will even ask us, "Is your Realtor meeting us here?" Evidently we pass as an odd couple with a wardrobe mismatch disorder.

Al takes command. "You must be Shelley. I'm Al, and this is my client, Kate." As I shake hands with the agent, I realize I know her from somewhere. It takes a circuit through the house and barn before it clicks into my brain: the Prodigal Son. She and her husband used to own a little coffeehouse by that name in Hyannis. They provided the venue for the monthly belly-dance extravaganza that my friend Katrina used to organize. Before we depart, I mention this connection.

"You used to dance, right?" Shelley asks.

"Kali was my dance name," I say with a smile. "Always a lot of veil work. Once I came close to taking out three pieces of art you were exhibiting on the wall behind the stage."

"I remember you." Shelley laughs and tells me she is happy being free of restaurant hours and looking forward to selling houses.

I think about telling her there is no chance in hell that I will buy this old house for which the seller is asking in excess of half a million dollars. It's gloomy, overfurnished, and needs a ton of work. The barn, where I had thought I might be able to create an office, would require a complete overhaul—electricity, plumbing, interior walls, heat. Another hundred grand. I don't say any of this to Shelley, but rather say that I am early in the process of looking for a place with enough space for my mother and me to live together and enough privacy for me to work without interruption.

"Sure," she says. "Well, good luck to you."

"And to you in your new career," I say before Al and I head back to his shiny truck, purchased to straddle his competing business interests: comfort and luxury for his real estate clients, and a big bed to haul all the equipment he needs for his landscaping customers.

"Nice truck," I say as we buckle up. "I could live in it."

✍

Between appointments we stop for lunch, eating bagel sandwiches off paper plates in a little joint in West Yarmouth. Al, suited for more formal fare, is by far the best-dressed and best-looking man in the Cape Cod winter sea of fleece and denim. Now that I've peeled back the puffy red parka, I look a bit more presentable, though still about two levels of formalwear shy of my luncheon companion. I think about this—why? Because if we were on a first date, I would be hoping for a second.

But we aren't dating. We are trying to figure out how I can take care of my mother and take care of myself at the same time. Over the past several months I've realized that the situation as it exists right now—two houses separated by a town line and about twenty minutes of driving time—is not working. My mother calls me several times a day with crises large and small. She loses her car keys routinely, occasionally her wallet. She telephones for help and, if she doesn't reach me, leaves this message: "Kate, this is your mother. Call me as soon as you get this."

"Mom," I ask her, "when you leave a message, could you say a bit about why you're calling? I worry something horrible has happened."

She seems to understand my request, but finds it impossible to honor.

If I don't respond right away, she will call again. And again. She gathers urgency, and sometimes irritation, with each repeat call. She doesn't believe that I cannot take her calls; rather, she thinks that I am avoiding her.

"Katie. Pick up the phone. Pick up. This is your mother. Pick up, goddamn it."

She fails to understand that she is talking into the void of voice mail, that even if I could pick up the phone, goddamn it, I can't hear her voice until I dial in for my messages.

I find the repeated phone calls difficult. My work often requires me to be on the office phone for long stretches at a time. When I hear the home phone ringing, I know it is likely to be my mother. I am learning that she is probably not in serious trouble, but there is some part of me that worries she could be. And so I am in equal measures worried, distracted while working, and annoyed that she is bothering me during my workday.

On days when the phone is quiet, it is usually because my mother is at her computer. I'll get off a client conference to discover more than a dozen e-mails, each rife with spelling errors that would have appalled my English-teacher mother as recently as a year ago. She blames "the typos" on the arthritis in her fingers, or on the keyboard, or on her computer; but as I read through her multiple misspellings, I realize that something serious is happening to my mother. She hasn't just forgotten how to spell some words. She has forgotten that spelling matters to her. She has forgotten who she is.

Or was.

In response, I take my mother grocery shopping. Once a week I drive over to her house and collect her for lunch and a spin around her local supermarket. I acquire the proper frequent shopper card, and sometimes we use it to take advantage of the sales. But mostly my mother wants to eat peanut butter and Ritz crackers and the occasional liverwurst sandwich. I try to buy the healthier brand of peanut butter, but that doesn't go over well. So I give in to Jif and Skippy and the high sugar content that can't be a boon to her already compromised health. The only advantage of my mother's limited diet: shopping is easy. I can breeze through the store—peanut butter, Ritz crackers, Maxwell House coffee, nondairy creamer, liverwurst, pumpernickel bread, Oreos, toilet paper, tissues. Before I pick up these necessities, I position my mother in the produce department with a shopping cart to support her as she moves slowly through the opening aisles of the store. I encourage her to put anything she wants into the cart. Usually she selects coffee cake or a Boston cream pie from the bakery department, but occasionally she takes home some seedless grapes or a bunch of bananas.

Some part of me believes that if I could fix my mother's diet, I could fix her mind. I know she eats a good dinner with Bill on Friday nights. I make a point to make sure she gets at least another lunch and dinner with me every week. When we're together, I watch her put away a ton of food. It isn't that she has lost her appetite. I send her home with leftovers, which she dutifully stores in the refrigerator, never to be touched again—until I throw them out a week later.

No longer cooking, I have been told, can be an early sign of dementia, but I'm not sure this is the best marker for my mother's mental capacity. She has never enjoyed cooking. Sure, Mom put meals on the table when I was growing up, but she passed that task to me as soon as I could handle an oven mitt. Her tendency not to cook is long-standing.

The year that my parents divorced, my mother and I ate a lot of Swanson's TV dinners. The foodie I've become is horrified by this fact, but the truth is, I loved sitting at the kitchen table with my mother, eating our hot-from-the-oven dinners out of shiny aluminum trays. Our regulars were turkey and fried chicken. I thought they were delicious. Both came with mashed potatoes and gravy; one with corn, one with green beans. I can't remember now which of the entrées featured the bubbling apple crisp for dessert, but that was my favorite. Sometimes my mother let me have hers too. We never cared much for the Swanson's Salisbury steak, but we were big fans of Dinty Moore beef stew. And not to forget Howard Johnson's frozen macaroni and cheese. It had those bread crumbs on top that made the cheese turn crispy orange. I loved HoJo's mac and cheese almost as much as the Kraft chicken noodle dinner that came in a box and required the use of a pot and the addition of water.

Remembering our frozen food days, I decide to stock my mother's freezer with the present-day equivalent. I read the labels carefully, avoiding the brands loaded with unpronounceable ingredients. I try to take into account my mother's taste and look for things I would never eat—like lobster bisque—but that I know she loves. Pleased with myself, I remind her that she only needs to open the freezer and pop dinner into the microwave, that she can have a decent hot meal in minutes.

She keeps eating peanut butter crackers and liverwurst sandwiches.

"Emily likes liverwurst," she says, and I imagine my mother sitting in her smoky den, watching TV and feeding scraps of stretchy meat to the small gray cat perched on the arm of her chair.

The smell, the texture, and the concept of liverwurst keep me far away from it. I wonder if it has any nutritional value whatsoever. At least a frozen entrée has a label on it that outlines what you're getting. I show my mother the crammed freezer and suggest that one of these dinners would make a nice change of pace for her. She agrees.

"Do you forget what's in there?" I ask, trying to understand why she hasn't touched the frozen food.

"Oh no. But I don't know what to do with them."

"What do you mean?" I ask.

"Well, could you show me how to cook one sometime?"

It had never occurred to me that my mother might not know how to cook a frozen dinner. I take one out of the freezer and consider: she probably can't read the small-print instructions without her glasses—which, along with the car keys, are routinely MIA. And if you can't read the instructions, you wouldn't know that sometimes you take off the overwrap and sometimes you just make one-inch slits in it before you put the tray into the microwave. And how would you know how many minutes to cook the thing if you couldn't read the directions on the package? If somehow you managed to figure all that out, removing the cellophane wouldn't be an easy task for arthritic hands and fingers.

I go over the basics with my mother, and I realize by the way she is paying attention that this isn't just about the miniscule printed instructions on the side of the package. She is having trouble following the directions, even if she can read them. And I think she's afraid of her microwave. She's forgotten how it works. What I don't understand yet is that she has lost at least some of her ability to sequence; she can no longer rely on her memory to help her perform a series of steps in order to complete a task.

I'd been thinking that if I went to my mother's house for dinner every so often, my presence might prompt her to prepare a hot meal. But the experience tonight makes it clear to me that neither a freezer full of frozen entrées nor hosting her only daughter at her dinner table will change my mother's eating habits.

The problem, I am starting to understand, is larger than getting in the groceries and coaxing my mother to eat, bigger than keeping her house clean and her trash taken away. I think about the wool socks I found "drying" in her oven. I consider her uncertain relationship with the microwave. I begin to wonder whether my mother is safe in her own home.

∽

That's why I called Al. That's how I became the equivalent of his first dollar bill.

Maybe we can find a duplex, or even better, two cottages on one property. I seek some perfect place that gives us each a sense of privacy and also a shared sense of security. In this fantasy, I cook meals for my mother. She gains weight and mental prowess through better nutrition. And she doesn't feel the need to call or e-mail several times a day, because she knows she'll see me every night for dinner. Sure, I am aware that my mother's health may continue to decline, even with a better living situation and regular meals; but I believe that maybe I can slow things down, make things better for her—and for me too.

In order to create this haven of shared meals and easy access, I will have to sell my place and my mother will have to sell hers. We'll still end up with a mortgage—possibly one that is larger than our combined debt now. A mortgage I won't be able to afford alone. Which means this imaginary shared property is a temporary solution that I will have to sell if my mother ends up needing more care. As I drive around with Al, looking at house after ineligible house, I consider whether my vision, if I can make it real, is the best of all possible plans.

I know my mother loves the place she calls her "wee cottage," and I'm awfully fond of my home too. I love the brick steps that lead to the front door. I love the deck that floats in the treetops. I love the colors inside and the animals outside. And my cat, Bix, loves our house too. He came to me only five months after my long-lived companion cat, Egypt, departed the planet. Bix claimed me—and my heart—long before I had planned to adopt another kitty. But cats have their own timing and their own agendas. We cat-appreciative humans are therefore capable of adaptation. I took in this beautiful Maine Coon, whose unfortunate shelter name was Todd. He'd come all the way from Georgia on the Petfinder network and had spent the last five months of his life living in one cage after another. When he laid eyes on me, he seemed to be saying, "Don't even talk to me unless you're planning to take me home." In fact, I talked to him for three consecutive days—over Memorial Day weekend—until the adoption was approved, and I petted him for the first time without bars between us.

Bix is on the "con" list I am making in my head, along with the house-love my mother and I share. Then there's the book.

In a few months' time, my publisher will be sending me on tour to promote the paperback of *Cottage for Sale*. Because I toured in New England for the hardcover, I already know some of the questions I can expect. Way up there on the list—right after the high level of interest in my current love life—readers want to know how it feels to live in my expanded home.

"Do you love it?" they ask me.

Always, I answer: "Yes, I do."

"Can you ever imagine moving?"

"I can't—or at least I wouldn't want to. It's perfect."

Well, that's the answer I had been giving. Only the truth.

I can hear the inevitable question on my upcoming tour: "How's the cottage?"

"On the market."

"I don't live there anymore."

"Sold."

It occurs to me that my integrity as a writer may require me to stay put a little while longer. But I don't mention this to Al as I climb out of his truck. I thank him for his time, his patience, his excellent advice, and also for lunch.

"Same time next week," he calls to me.

I give him an affirmative nod, a quick wave, and a smile. Then I climb into my car and head home.

Chapter Five

Smoking

My mother is a smoker. Not the kind of smoker who wants to quit, or even the kind who tries to quit and cannot, but the kind of smoker who is offended by nonsmoking sections and no-smoking signs. She thinks the concept of secondhand smoke was invented by a bunch of ex-smokers. "People who give up smoking have such a holier-than-thou attitude. The truth is, they don't want to inhale secondhand smoke because it reminds them of how great it was when they used to light up." My mom is the kind of smoker who, despite her lifelong liberal leanings, sounds a lot like a libertarian when she talks about how the government shouldn't be interfering with a citizen's right to smoke. My mother is an unrepentant, unapologetic, and unceasing smoker. She has smoked as long as I have been alive. And then some.

When pressed, she attributes her smoking to my father's influence. "It was self-defense," she has told me more than once, describing her unhappy life as a young navy wife in Key West, the mandatory dinner parties, the feeling that she didn't fit in. "Your father smoked, all the other officers and their wives smoked. I figured if I can't beat 'em, I better join 'em."

And join 'em she did—never looking back and never seeming to regret her decision. My father, the alleged impetus for the smoking habit, was not the dedicated smoker that my mother became. I don't recall his brand—perhaps because he was more a bummer than a buyer of tobacco products—though I believe his preferred pack was a crimson color with white lettering. Around the time my father remarried, he quit smoking.

It is said that the universe abhors a vacuum. My mother was happy to fill this one by producing just that much more poisonous air.

My mother smokes Benson & Hedges Lights. The package is gold. The lettering is maroon and black. And the little cellophane pull-open strip is shiny gold. When I was a kid, she would send me in to pick up a pack, offering a bribe to get me to run in—enough extra cash for a Milky Way or a Three Musketeers bar. In those days, knowing that the smoking parent was waiting in the car, the cashier would hand over the cigarettes and a complimentary matchbook to my thirteen-year-old self.

For years and years of my life—even before she asked me to secure her cigarettes—I tried to persuade my mother to quit smoking.

"You have asthma!" I would say. "How can you even inhale?" Asthmatic myself, I couldn't imagine how she could breathe smoke into her already fragile respiratory system. Though my question was not rhetorical, my mother chose never to answer it. She just kept smoking.

"It's not good for me to be around you smoking!" Guilt-tripping was likewise ineffective. I tried scare tactics, informational lectures, all the usual methods. Nothing worked.

"I enjoy smoking," my mother would say. "Just allow me that. Do I ask you to stop doing the things you enjoy?"

"But this is about your health—"

"Exactly. *My* health. Stop nagging me, Katie."

In time—maybe fifteen years ago—I did as she asked. I

realized that nothing I could do or say would alter my mother's allegiance to her smoking ways. I asked her not to smoke in my home or in my car, and she came to terms with my terms. A truce was achieved. We make multiple stops whenever we take a long journey together, and I keep an ashtray tucked under the bench in the front garden.

At her house, I have little or no say in my mother's inclination to light up. Most of the time she will oblige me if I ask her not to smoke. But when she isn't smoking in the present moment, the smoke of cigarettes past still hangs in the air. That's why I spend more time here in the warmer months, when the windows can be opened. The summer is the easiest time of year for my breathing and, I've decided, the best time for me to make a dent in the unopened mail that Noelle has stacked in my mother's living room. After we unload the groceries, I dive in.

"Let's open the mail, Ma."

"Oh, let's just have some of those brownies. Do you want ice cream?"

"C'mon, Mom, we have to get a look at what's here."

"Why bother? Ice cream?" she persists.

"No, thanks. I'll wait till later. I'm going to start without you, then."

"Kathleen! That is *my mail!*"

"And you've been refusing to open it for months, so I can't believe you're that attached to it."

She can't help but laugh, even as she thinks to remind me that mail tampering is a federal offense. Her comment reminds me of the arguments I had with my first best friend, Bobby: "Do you want to make a federal case out of it?" I'm not sure where we picked up that line, but we used it on each other with some frequency.

"Report me," I say now.

She sits down on the couch, balancing her plate on her lap because the table in front of her is covered in mail.

"See—it's in your way. Let's just do this. Clear it out. You'll feel so much better. Do you have a trash bag?"

She directs me to a carton of Hefty bags. I begin to open the mail in no particular order, and I realize my mother has done some sorting of her own. There are no catalogs or flyers in this mail, no bulk mail or requests for donations.

"Yes, just bills," my mother agrees.

"Mom, if you don't open your mail, how do you know when to pay these?" I am swimming in mail that dates back more than two years.

"Oh, if they want the money, they'll call me. I just pay over the phone."

After a while, I start checking postmarks rather than taking the time to open everything. I make rules: Envelopes with postmarks prior to 2003—two years ago—will be tossed, unopened. Mail that is postmarked between one and two years ago will be opened and stacked for later review. I set aside anything less than a year old for priority handling. In this multiyear mother lode of ignored missives are the bills for all her utilities, for her Sears charge; notices from Medicare, from her insurance company, from the Registry of Motor Vehicles. There are collections notices, shutoff notices, and more than one threatening letter.

As I sort, scan, and read, I do my best to appear unruffled. In truth, I am frightened by what I have uncovered. My mother hasn't paid her Medicare premium in at least a year. She is driving an unregistered vehicle that is possibly uninsured and no doubt uninspected.

"What about the mortgage?" I haven't seen a bill, but I haven't seen any threats from the mortgage company either.

"Oh, the bank pays that."

"What do you mean?"

"You know—the bank takes it right out of my check every month."

Thank God for small favors.

"Mom, if it's okay with you, I'm going to take your mail home with me. I think there are some problems we need to solve—like with your Medicare—"

"Don't tell me about the damn Medicare! They don't pay anything! All I get is notices—they don't pay this and they don't pay that! Ever since I turned sixty-five!"

"Well, I'm not sure you even have Medicare anymore—"

"And good riddance to them!"

"Yeah. I'm going to take these stacks home and sort them in my office. It will be easier there. We'll go over everything together next week, okay?"

"If you want my bills, my darling daughter, you are welcome to them. Feel free to pay them, too. How about a brownie?"

This time I accept the offer.

∽

On my way home, I can smell the bills. Literally. They have been sitting around my mother's house for so long that they are infused with stale cigarette smell. Damn her smoking. It makes everything that much more challenging. I'm thinking about the house hunt, which has been temporarily suspended while I re-group and rethink what might be best.

I'm still in regular touch with Al, and we speak often enough that I recognize his cell phone number when it pops up without his name on caller ID.

"Really," he said recently, "the smartest thing would be to

sell your mom's house and use that money to add on to your house, so your mother could come live with you."

It isn't that I haven't thought about that—hard. Before I added on the cottage to create my office space, I lived and worked in three rooms. It was a tight squeeze that resulted in office equipment in the kitchen and file cabinets in my bedroom closet, but I managed for eleven years. For most of that time I lived only with my cat, Egypt. But for fourteen months in the mid-1990s, my living room became my mother's bedroom. I bought a futon couch so she would have a comfortable place to sleep. I cleared out the living room closet, and we organized some bins around the fireplace for her stuff. The kitchen separated my bedroom/office from my mother's room, and it was during this period that I became obsessive about keeping the kitchen island clear. That six-foot by two-foot expanse in the neutral zone seemed to hold the key to my sanity.

When my mother came to live with me, she was just out of rehab. I took it as a good sign that she had no desire to return to her house—the place I thought of as the scene of the crime, even if all evidence had been cleared by the disaster cleanup company. It was always more house than she could afford in retirement. We were pretty sure she would lose money on the sale, but it seemed clear to both of us—and to my uncle Jack, who was, and is, my principal adviser on all things Mom—that the only option was to try to sell the place, bad market or not. In the meantime, she would move in with me.

My mother bemoaned the lack of television in my house, and she listened to the radio almost constantly. While I made dinner, we listened together to *All Things Considered* on the kitchen speakers; but while I was working, my mother tuned in to Rush Limbaugh and G. Gordon Liddy on the smaller radio she kept on a windowsill in the living room. This was during the Clinton era, when the rhetoric of the Republican right was at an all-time inflammatory high. I'd only need to catch a phrase here or there and I would get all worked up. More than once I wanted to hurl the radio through the living room window. But I couldn't give Rush or the man I thought of as Watergate Liddy the satisfaction. "Don't people care that guy is a crook?"

My mother, the woman who routinely wrote to Ted Kennedy when she saw a social injustice to be righted, only laughed.

"Seriously, how can you listen to this vitriol?"

"You have to know what they're thinking."

At night, the same station featured Dr. Laura Schlessinger giving relationship advice. Long after my mother had conked out for the night, I could hear the distraught husbands and wives, girlfriends and boyfriends tell their desperate stories of love and sex gone wrong. When I knew my mother was sound asleep, I would tiptoe into the living room to turn off the radio. But sometimes I listened to Dr. Laura while I puttered in the kitchen, half of me fascinated and half of me horrified by the questions and answers I heard.

"She's harsh," I said to my mother one evening when Dr. Laura's show came on.

"She is," my mother said, "but she's smart."

But not as smart as my mother. After ten months on the market, her house sold, predictably, at a loss. The bank accepted the short sale, and my mother walked away with nothing. We sold a lot of her larger furniture to a dealer who came to the house with cash and a truck. The rest of it we moved to a large, sunny second-floor apartment a town away. My mother lived there for a year before she decided to go house hunting again. The real estate crisis that had caused her to lose her shirt meant there were opportunities out there.

"I want a little cottage like yours," she announced. We checked out many possibilities before she found the one she lives in now. The septic system failed inspection, the roof had noticeable bald spots, and it wasn't the cleanest place we'd seen. But my mother liked the idea of being close to a lake, away from the main drag. She managed to buy the place for seventy-five thousand dollars and no money down, with the seller assuming the costs of the necessary repairs. I was impressed with my mother for her persistence and her real estate savvy. In a little more than two years she had gotten sober, stayed sober, and turned the loss of her not inconsiderable investment in one too-big house into an affordable mortgage on a little cottage that was just right.

For the fourteen months that we shared our living quarters, my mother got into the habit of stepping outside for a smoke. I felt guilty sending her outdoors in the winter months, but for the sake of my own health, I enforced the rules we'd agreed upon. Whenever I consider the idea of living with my mother again, I get stuck on the smoking issue. This time, she would be moving into more than a temporary resting place. If I dictate what she can and cannot do, how will she think of my house—or any place we live—as her home? And if I don't make rules around the smoking, how can I live—and breathe—in the same space?

Back at my house, I leave the bag of bills on the deck to air out, and I call Al. "What about a condo?" I ask him. "Close to me, but a space of her own?"

"Well, the condo market is slipping, but they still aren't cheap. It's possible we could find something close to you for about the same price we would get for her house. But then you'd have the mortgage plus condo fees."

"Yeah, I know. But can we check some out?"

"Sure," he says. "I'll send you some listings later today."

⌒

"A condo?" my uncle Jack says when we speak later that week. "Why not an apartment? If she sold her house, she'd have enough money to rent a nice apartment. She wouldn't have to worry about anything. And you wouldn't have to sell it when she needs more care."

Jack has been lobbying for my mother to move into a senior living apartment. It isn't that I think it's a bad idea, but I don't know how to sell my mother on it. "You want me to go live with a bunch of old people?" she asked me when I mentioned she might enjoy living in a less isolated setting with more retired people around.

"A condo, because she has a cat and she's a smoker. I've been watching apartment ads. Hardly any allow pets, and lots are advertising for nonsmoking tenants. Insurance, I guess."

"Have you spoken to her about putting her house on the market?" he asks me.

"Not in detail. I've mentioned it might be better if she lived closer to me. She said that sounded nice, but that she didn't like the idea of moving again. I told her not to worry, we'd figure it out together, and I'd be there to help. But first I need to understand what's out there for her."

"But you'll have to sell her place to buy a condo."

"Yes," I say. "We will."

"Have you talked to Bill lately?" he asks.

"No. They've been over for dinner a few times, but I haven't talked to him alone since our chat."

Bill and I had met for lunch around the time I began house hunting with Al. I told him, in the gentlest terms, that I was worried about Mom's living alone.

"Your mother's health insurance is all screwed up," he said. "You need to look into that. She should have Medicare plus a supplement. And I don't think she's going for her checkups, because she says her insurance doesn't cover anything. I'm concerned about that." He talked about his supplementary insurance and told me he'd be glad to give me more information in case she needed a new policy.

"Thanks," I said. "I'll look into that." Trying to steer the conversation back to my mother's possible relocation, I told him about a colonial duplex I'd found a few towns away.

"It sounds ideal," he offered.

"In some ways, yes, but I know you work, and it might be harder to get together with Mom on the weekends if she were further away."

He said nothing. He returned to the topic of her health care for a few minutes before telling me he'd applied for a couple of jobs. "Off-Cape," he said. "I'd have mixed feelings about moving if I got an offer, but I'd consider it."

It was my turn to be silent. It wasn't that I thought Bill would come to the rescue, pledge his undying loyalty to my mother, and suggest they move in together, but I guess I was hoping to hear that my mother and I were not in this alone. With his job-hunting announcement, my mother's companion let me know he was uninterested in making any kind of commitment to the woman he'd been not-dating for three-plus years now.

"Do you think he's backing off?" Jack asks me.

"Maybe."

"That would be a real shame. He's the only regular social contact she has, outside of you."

∽

A few weeks after the mail retrieval and before I have her finances sorted out, my mother calls. "Bill dumped me," she says.

"What?"

"He dumped me. And the worst of it is, he didn't even have the spine to tell me to my face. He wrote me a letter. Typed! Can you believe that? I thought he was a gentleman."

"Let's go to lunch," I suggest. "I'll be there in an hour."

At her house, my mother shows me the letter—typed on his computer and printed on cheap paper. It says he feels like he and my mother have less and less to talk about. He has met a woman in a class he is taking, and he wants to be free to pursue a friendship with her. He wishes my mother well. It is short, sweet, and devoid of any lingering affection.

"Maybe he was too scared to tell you in person," I say.

"The coward!" my mother hisses.

"Yeah. This just sucks, Mom. I'm really sorry."

For once, she does not tell me that ladies do not talk about things sucking. She agrees: "It does suck."

Over lunch, we are just two women, puzzled and hurt by the ways of men. And angry. She's mad as hell about the way he broke it off.

"We were friends," she says. "We weren't romantic. Why does he have to dump his friend just so he can be friends with this . . . *chicky* in his class?"

"Excellent point," I say. "Obviously he thought you were more than friends."

"Well, not anymore. We're nothing now."

We stop on the way back to my mother's house so she can buy a carton of cigarettes. I can't say I blame her for wanting to lay in the supplies. She will be smoking and stewing over this for some time to come. I suggest she rip up the note, or burn it, or do something cathartic with it, but she wants to hold on to it for now. "I just may write the bastard back."

Driving back to my place, I consider that my mother's mind

was not the least bit cloudy today. She didn't repeat herself or forget for one minute what Bill had done. But I also wonder if the reason Bill wrote to her was because he thought she might not remember what he told her in a conversation. Or even that he'd already told her this in person, but she had forgotten. That he felt he had to write it down for her. I argue with myself over this, deciding that even if he had tried to tell her in person, he could have handled this differently. He could have, for one thing, given me some warning. I've always liked Bill, and I feel hurt not only on my mother's behalf. For almost four years, Bill has been a part of birthday celebrations, family gatherings, holidays. No more. Like my mother said, "We're nothing now."

Even while I'm cursing Bill for his awkward and cowardly breakup methods and the way he has hurt my mother, I realize that, in a perverse way, he's done me a favor. Now I have no worries about moving Mom too far away from her gentleman companion.

I stay close to my mother for the next several days, concerned that she will become depressed. "A letter typed on his computer!" she says again and again, but this, it seems to me, is the kind of deconstructive repetitiveness we all engage in when something or someone has hurt us.

"Maybe now would be a good time to make a move," I suggest one late afternoon. We are sitting at her kitchen table, which, thanks to Noelle, is clear and clean.

"Get the hell out of Dodge," my mother says.

"Why don't I invite Al over to talk about putting your place on the market?"

"What would Al know about it?"

"He's a real estate guy now—remember I told you?"

"Oh, right. Does he know anything?"

"Well, he had to take courses. And if you decided to sell, you'd be helping him out with his first commission." My mother has a soft spot for Al. They have long chats whenever he mows her lawn.

"It won't sell till the spring," she says. "And what would I do with my stuff? Where would I go?"

"We'll take it one step at a time. Shall I call Al?"

"Sure," she says. "What the hell. Call Al. Do you mind if I have a cigarette?"

Chapter Six

Mother-Daughter

I am a daughter who has become a mother. Not in the usual way. I have no children of my own. I am mother to my mother.

In the manner of a modern parent—and long before this summer, when I arranged to receive her mail and to pay her bills—I have worked to keep my mother's life in order. I learned to make breakfast using the kitchen stepstool to reach the toaster, and I can recall doing my best to distract my mother on the nights when my father didn't show up for dinner. But I saw my mother's need for protection most clearly when my parents separated. Broken up and literally made ill by my parents' lost marriage, I took on the care of my mom—willingly and without regret. At the ripe old age of ten, I thought of my childhood as something that had kept me occupied between the ages of three and nine.

Not that things were exactly idyllic in that six-year span. My father worked hard and played harder. He had a bad habit of gambling away the mortgage money. To make ends meet, my mother started subbing at the elementary school. Within a few years she earned her teaching certificate and took a full-time job at the high school. She was a gifted teacher, and she took pleasure in her students. But she resented my father and his un-reliability as a husband and provider. For my part, I wished my mother were like the neighbor ladies who stayed home, drank coffee, and greeted their children with fresh-baked cookies after school. My father, too, wished for a wife who stayed at home. He hated my mother's working—perhaps because he hated himself and the habit that forced his wife to cover his losses.

I was too young to know the truth of my parents' marriage or its ending. My mother's version of the events varied depending on her mood: my father asked for a divorce because he no longer wanted the responsibility of a family; my father asked for a divorce because he wanted to protect us from the loan sharks who were beginning to threaten us. My mother, at least in her own mind, never wanted to end the marriage. It was either her husband's desire—what could she do?—or the difficult but safe choice her husband told her they must make—and what could she do?

My mother, strong and courageous in her working life, was strangely passive in her personal relationships. I sensed her vulnerability and met it with a premature, role-reversed determination to keep her safe from harm.

I did my best to protect my mother, but there is only so much a kid can do—whether she is three or ten or thirteen and wishing like hell that her mother won't actually say *I do* to the man standing beside her at the altar in an old stone church. My mother wore cornflower blue; my aunt Rosemary, her maid of honor, was in navy. My uncles Bob and Jack wore dark suits. The few photographs taken that day confirm I wasn't the only one wishing my mother would have a last-minute change of heart. The groom looks ruddy and cheerful, but no one else is smiling—not the brothers or the sister or the bride's daughter or even the bride. In the photos we appear nervous, haunted, puzzled, scared, and sad. Emotions, it turned out, that were entirely appropriate.

My mother's second husband was tall, handsome, and capable of charming the grownups. But with the x-ray vision of a child, I saw trouble the first time I laid eyes on the man. I hoped against hope that my mother would come to her senses, stop seeing him, call off the wedding—or later, leave him. But she didn't. Not for many years.

Living with Richard, for me, was like living atop a live volcano. An eruption could occur at any time. I could try to outrun it, but ultimately the volcano was bigger than I was, with the potential to cause injury and harm. I moved through those years in a high state of anxiety, operating on minimal sleep, ever watchful. Some nights were peaceful. Many nights were not. They blur now in memory, but one stands out. I was a teenager. It was before I could drive, and I knew I needed to get my mother and myself out of the house. I began inching toward the phone in the living room.

"Go ahead," Richard taunted me, "call your father—*tell on me*—do you think he gives a shit about you? Go ahead—call him. He won't come."

"He will," I said, surprised I could even speak as Richard—heavy on his feet—moved closer to me, grabbing the telephone from my hands.

"Oh yeah? You think he'll come? Your father couldn't give a shit. If you are so sure he'll come rescue you, call him."

I was pressed up against the wall. Richard was way too close for comfort. He'd put down the phone—a chocolate-brown Trimline model that I own to this day—and both of his hands were free. I could feel it in him: he wanted to hit me, and hit me hard.

My mother—where was she? Across the room? Crying? Saying, *Richard, don't?* I don't recall for sure.

"Give me the phone and I'll call him right now," I said.

When I think back to that moment, I can't believe I dared to speak in such a volatile and scary situation. My tone, my absolute (and absolutely false) calm, stopped the blow that was building in him. He couldn't resist rising to my challenge. He reached for the phone, pushed it at me.

"Dial," he said, his face close to mine. I dialed. My father answered.

"Please come," I said. Did my father reply? I don't remember. I know I hung up and said to Richard, "He's coming. I'm meeting him at the Superette. I have to go now. Mom, I need a ride."

Richard, strangely subdued, allowed us to leave.

My mother drove to the dark convenience store parking lot, where we sat in a cold car waiting for my dad to drive the seventy miles between us, which he managed to do in about forty-five minutes. In the meantime, a cop pulled up to the car and told us that my father had called him.

"Should I go check on the house?" he asked my mother. Somehow she persuaded him that all was okay, that her daughter and her new husband weren't getting along right now, no big deal.

But it was a big deal. After my father picked me up, my mother drove to Boston, to her sister's house. This I learned only recently from my aunt Rosemary.

"You haven't had an easy time, Katie."

Rose and I were on the phone; I was updating her on my progress with my mother's finances, health care, and housing. Somehow the conversation had turned to my childhood, to my mother's second husband. "She came here that night," Rosie said. "I'll never forget it."

It was long before cell phones, and my mother hadn't been able to call ahead. She just turned up on her younger sister's doorstep in the middle of the night. "She looked terrible. She was crying and trying to tell me what happened, and she had a bruise on the side of her face. She never said, but I'm pretty sure he hit her."

When Rosemary told me this, I felt like someone was hitting me. My mother had gone to her sister's house, had revealed the dirty secret of her second marriage in an undeniable way; and yet she returned, ultimately, to Richard, to her own personal hell—and mine. Sure, he made all sorts of promises: he loved my mother, he would change for her. My mother returned, and I came back a few days later—not because I believed that Richard would change, but rather because I feared he would not.

For the week or so that I lived with my father, I felt like part of a real family. My father brought a stability to his second marriage that he had never achieved in his first. He was a reliable provider with a stay-at-home wife and four children. Not only did he make it home in time for dinner; he bragged about his wife Theresa's cooking, jumped to clear the table, and did the dishes. Theresa found clothes for me to wear—some sweet little cardigans and jeans that had once been hers. "I used to be a lot skinnier," she joked. She took me to buy underwear and some basic essentials, and we had conversations about where I might live. She told me she hoped I might decide to stay. I felt welcome and cared for; I was tempted to relax and settle in. But I could not leave my mother alone to deal with Richard. I was sure that if I had not been there, my mother would have been unable to leave on her own. There was something missing in my mother, some instinct of self-preservation she lacked. I felt obliged to keep us as safe as we could be in a fundamentally unsafe environment.

For me, that meant keeping a low profile and doing as I was told. Richard said I was old enough to contribute to the household. As soon as I turned fourteen, I got my work permit and an after-school job at the public library. When I got home from the library, I performed my assigned chores, hoping to pass Richard's grim inspections of the bathroom, kitchen, den, living room. I did the laundry, prepared meals, and made sure I got good grades. I rarely slept—I felt compelled to stay awake until the wee hours of the morning, until I knew that Richard was sound asleep, until I felt sure that the threat, for that day, had passed. I never told a soul what was going on at home.

I spent every untormented moment practicing my flute. My guilty concern for my mother wasn't the only reason I returned home. I returned to my flute and to the band director who had become my musical mentor. I believed that music was my calling, my life, and my one-way ticket out. I wanted to take my mother with me the way I had that night—and the many nights, after I got my driver's license, when I hustled her into the car and drove us to safety. But I was beginning to understand that my mother wasn't going anywhere, not for a while, and not for long. I also knew that Richard hated having me around. Part of me believed that things between them might improve if I left for college, and another part of me was beginning to understand that I had to save my own life before I could save my mother's.

I did go off to college—to a campus I had never seen, nestled in a town in upstate Ohio, an area known for minimal winter sunshine and endless lake-effect snow (weather that was unadvertised in the recruitment materials). While I was at school, my mother found her way out of her second marriage. To this day she has never shared the details of that achievement with me. She walked away from that life atop the volcano and bought two condos side by side, installing my grandmother in one, herself in the other. She adopted a poodle and named him Patrick. She purchased a piano. That summer, when I returned from school, there was little discussion of Richard or the seven-year reign of terror. That's when my mother began listening to the radio late at night: WBZ's Larry Glick and his wacky songs, strange guests, and my favorite feature, *The Story Behind the Story*. I remember listening that summer to the late-night radio coming from my mother's room and feeling like I'd won some giant jackpot: freedom from fear, freedom to sleep at night.

∾

Now that I have made my way through the Hefty bag of unopened mail, I understand that my mother, by not paying so many bills, has accumulated over seven thousand dollars in her checking account. An unorthodox savings method, for sure, but having a chunk of change in her account enables me to get things up to date. I pay off her Sears charge—including the 24 percent interest they have been throwing at her every month—and close the account. I renew her car insurance—they make us pay a whole year's premium up front because the policy has lapsed. We get the car registered and inspected. I will spend hours on the phone and online, write letters, fill out reams of paperwork, and visit the Social Security office on her behalf to solve the mystery of her missing health insurance, to find an interim solution, and eventually to reinstate her Medicare coverage.

Sometimes my mother resists my interventions, and sometimes I resent the time I am giving over to the care and maintenance of her life's business. I almost wonder whether she has created this mess on purpose—to rope me in, to be rescued by me.

"You're always so organized, Katie," she has said to me through the years. The way she says the word, *organized*, it sounds like it is a quality that detracts from my personality. As if by being organized I have given up being creative or interesting or lively or fun. Just last week, sealing up a letter—my third—requesting interim health insurance and showing proof of noncoverage, I thought, *maybe she just prefers chaos.*

There are moments when I feel trapped, annoyed, and angry, even as I forge ahead, trying to straighten out what seems to be a giant mess of my mother's own making. I've been thrust into the role of parent—*organized* parent—again. I find myself remembering fondly a period only a few years ago—the period after my mother stopped drinking and when she was content in her cottage. We would meet for lunch and go shopping together. We talked on the phone and spent holidays together. We went to plays. For maybe the first time in our lives, we were mother-daughter, not daughter-mother, and we were, it turned out, great together. But now? We seem to be back where we started, when I was ten—or maybe even, as my mother claims, when I was three. I'm bossy and not always kind. I get the work done, but not always gracefully. I'm unhappy in the reprise of this role reversal. Maybe that's why I've been thinking about our life with Richard.

I have done my time in therapy, and I have spent hours in rooms with other adult children of alcoholics in an effort to understand and move beyond the influence of my mother's second husband. My mother, in contrast, has spared little thought for him. "I'm erasing that period," my mother told me years ago, when I discovered that she answered *widowed* rather than *divorced* when asked her marital status.

At first this bothered me. To deny that time was to deny the reality of my suffering and hers. Maybe because I still held her responsible—she was the grown-up, after all, who should have known better—I didn't want to let her off the hook so easily. Then there was the fact that my mother had been divorced from my father for fourteen years when he died. Theresa was his widow.

Over time, and as the shadow of my mother's second husband has diminished in my own life, I have begun to see some wisdom in my mother's revisionist history. Recently, I filled out a medical form on her behalf. I stared at the options only for a moment before I circled *W* for widowed.

It was only a few days after I circled that first *W* that someone asked me for the one word I would like people to use when they describe me after I die. I thought for only a few seconds before I answered, "Compassionate." There were all sorts of other words I could have chosen, words that said something about me, maybe about my writing, but those words flashed right by and the word *compassionate* came out. In the nanoseconds before I spoke the word aloud, I realized I was asking for help. To achieve that label in death, I would need to open my heart to my mother's need, right here, right now. And maybe I would need to exercise compassion toward myself—to cut myself a break for feeling angry and disappointed by the arc of the story of my mother and me. But I didn't think of that wrinkle on compassion when I answered the question. In that moment, I was only hoping I would have the strength, humor, goodwill, and empathy to move through this next phase of daughter-mother, mother-daughter.

Chapter Seven

Don't Get Old

It's the third Monday in September, and I'm hosting butter-flies. My prerehearsal anxiety is a relic, an excavated shard of remembrance: freshman year and a conservatory curriculum. Music theory classes, piano "individuals," juried performances, and a flute teacher who did not waste her time telling me when I played a passage well. Dig even deeper: high school band, an-other freshman year. A band director with high expectations and a harsh temper. Red-faced, threatening, stopping the band, index finger pointed at me. "No wonder you can't play the part! You don't even know how to put your flute together!" All eyes on me, my face now as red as his. "Ellen, fix it," he said, spitting his words at the senior who occupied the first chair.

In fact, I did not have the three pieces of my flute in correct alignment on that high school afternoon. If you could draw an imaginary line through the center of the flute's mouthpiece, I learned that day, it would bisect the keys on the middle section of the flute and run right along the rod on the foot joint. My ignorance, though inexcusable, was explicable. I'd learned how to play flute from brass-playing band directors. And my flute playing was inspired not by my passion but rather by the words of a pediatric specialist: "Allergy shots might help, and so would playing a wind instrument."

"A wind instrument?" my mother had repeated.

"Playing a wind instrument regulates breathing and builds lung capacity," the doctor told my mother.

His name was Dr. MacLean. I remember liking him better than his partner in practice, whose only advice to my mother had been "Get rid of the dogs."

I'd met Dr. MacLean's partner at Cardinal Cushing Hospital, where he'd shot me up with adrenaline and confirmed that the horrible chest colds I'd been having since I was a toddler were asthma attacks. He sent me to Children's Hospital in Boston, where I found the staff more sympathetic—though perhaps they were just expecting me. After administering another shot of adrenaline, the doctor asked if I thought I could swallow a pill. My memory of that process—the nurse handing me a Dixie cup first, then the pill in a little paper holder like the kind they use to serve catsup at roadside burger joints—remains vivid to this day. I was struggling for breath—years later, my mother told me I was struggling for life that night—and I was a willing patient, willing to swallow anything I could in the hope that I would once more be able to do what we tend to take for granted: inhale and exhale.

It would be several weeks of supervised recovery before I would meet Dr. MacLean, before he would suggest, in the same sentence, a regimen of allergy shots and a wind instrument. My mother acted on the doctor's recommendation when the new school year began.

"Have you decided which instrument you want to play?"

I remember the question. I remember my mother, pausing at the door of my bedroom just before she left for the evening meeting where she would rent me an instrument.

"Clarinet," I answered.

She smiled, and returned home two hours later with a flute.

"I think you'll like it better," she said. Even then, I knew that what she really was saying was that *she* liked it better. I was disappointed. Playing the clarinet would have meant sitting next to my friend Debbie, who also played clarinet. And playing the clarinet would have meant I could have asked my dad for tips. He hadn't played in years, but I remembered how upset he was when he discovered that my grandmother—well-meaning and ill-informed as to the ways of musical instruments—had given his silver clarinet a good, soapy soak. The pads were swollen, the instrument unplayable, my father sad and disbelieving.

Instead, I was presented with a flute. It wasn't what I wanted, and I was annoyed at my mother for foisting her preference on me. Still, I opened up the forest-green plastic case, lined with black velvet and containing three pieces of what would be assembled into my first flute. Shiny, silver—in fact, it was made of polished nickel—and complicated. Those were my first impressions. I hadn't a clue how to put it together or even how to make a basic sound. Neither did my mother. We just stared at it.

"It's prettier than a clarinet," my mother said.

✍

On my way to rehearsal tonight, my mother's situation is in the forefront of my mind. I'm working on persuading her that we need to put her house up for sale. She's not against it, but she's having a hard time imagining where she would go. I'm keeping that vague. "Closer to me," I've said.

"I'd like to be closer to you. That would be good."

That's one response. An hour later she might say, "But I love my wee little cottage. I don't want to go anywhere."

We'd cycle through it again—my reasoning, which I limit to keeping her safe and making it easier for us to visit; her agreement, and soon thereafter, her refusal to move. Sometimes the refusal is more emphatic than the agreement: "Who the hell put you in charge of me?"

My mother. If not for my mother, I would be hauling a clarinet to this rehearsal. *It's prettier.* Of all the inane reasons to pick an instrument. I smile, remembering our first sight of the instrument that would become mine. My mother selected the flute for me for all the wrong reasons, but I cannot deny she made the right choice.

∽

"Don't get old, Katie, don't get old." My mother has been saying that a lot lately. She says it when her arthritis makes it impossible for her to complete a simple task, but also in those moments when she realizes she has forgotten a conversation we have had.

"Mom, remember we talked about—"

"No, I don't remember. I can't remember what I had for breakfast, for Pete's sake." She shakes her head, considering her incapacity, and gives me this advice: "Don't get old."

"Consider the alternative," I offer her in turn, and she concedes that living is better than not. Still, I think about what she is saying—and not saying. The part of me that feels young, and that thinks of my mother—she just turned sixty-nine—as still relatively young in the grand scheme of things, believes that being alive is better than being dead. But another part of me, the part that knows we are both aging, ponders what it means to grow old. I think of my grandmother—Nana, my mother's mother. She aged gracefully, working as executive secretary to the planning board until she was required by city ordinance to retire at age seventy. In her early retirement, she was healthy, strong, and always on the move. When I picture her, I see her walking. A city dweller for most of her life, Nana never learned to drive a car. She was short—maybe five-three with her shoes on. I had at least five inches on her, but she could outpace my long-legged youth.

Maybe eight or nine years into her retirement, my grandmother began to show signs of dementia—or senility, as they called it then. While my mother and her siblings were coping with the changes in their mother's behavior, I was away at college and then setting out on my own. I never gave her condition much thought—eighty seems ancient from the perspective of your teens and twenties. I thought senility was an inevitability that accompanied growing *really* old. But I remember thinking, even way back then, that my grandmother was sharp as a whip while she was still working.

So was my mother. Is her early debility connected to her early retirement? Is this a possibly genetic tendency toward dementia, or a possibly genetic inability to cope with unstructured time? Jack, several years my mother's senior, keeps up a consulting practice in his semiretirement, and Rosemary, a few years younger, continues to work as a contractor for General Electric. Connection or coincidence? Do my aunt and uncle ever worry what they might forget if they stop showing up for work?

And me? I'm thinking there may be an upside to an inadequate retirement fund. Maybe—if I work until I drop—I can outfox the mind-muddling monster swimming in my gene pool.

∽

I thank Carol, the band librarian, as she hands me my folder before I make my way to the front of the band. Passing behind her seat, I say hello to Deb, our lead trumpet. She's unpacking her gear. I see that Bob, the principal clarinet and possibly my favorite person in the band, is already seated and warming up. Sometimes the solo players on flute and clarinet share a phrase, and through years of playing together, we listen and meld our voices almost as one. Bob plays with a depth of tone, a maturity, that I love to hear—a maturity that comes from playing an instrument for maybe sixty or seventy years of his life. He has survived colon cancer and a horrific back surgery. He needs a cane to get from his car to the rehearsal room. Sometimes he asks me to hold down the chair in front of him so he can lean on it to rise from the chair he's in. He never asks me to carry his music or his clarinet, but especially in the wintertime, I try to grab one or the other so he can focus on keeping his balance as we walk out to the parking lot.

Bob is almost ten years older than my mother, and I am pretty sure he would prefer aging to the alternative. It isn't that he's had an easy time of it, but he still wants to show up every week. For band and for life. After I greet my fellow flute players, I flash a smile in Bob's direction, and he gives me a nod and a grin before he returns to warming up his instrument, flipping through the folder on his music stand, anticipating what John has in store for us.

I do the same, coaxing my flute from the lowest tones of its range. Waking it slowly.

John welcomes us back, and we begin with a tone studies exercise before we do a quick tuning. Because we are associated with the Cape Cod Conservatory, our band is dedicated to learning new music every season. Our music library is not unlimited, so we do repeat selections—generally on programs that are years apart—but most of the music we will read tonight will be music we haven't seen before.

In our folders for December's concert are two operatic excerpts transcribed for wind ensemble, a medley of tunes from the Broadway musical *Oliver*, and a sprinkling of nontraditional holiday music, including one piece called *Russian Christmas Music*. Also programmed for December are two lesser-known marches, one by John Philip Sousa and one by British composer Kenneth Alford.

Tonight we'll play each selection from start to finish without stopping so that we get a sense of how the music is supposed to sound. Next week, John will begin to break each piece down into sections, drilling and refining before we reassemble the music in time for the concert seven weeks from now. But tonight we will just read. On the first rehearsal of the season, I don't worry about blowing a solo. All is forgiven—it's sight-reading, after all. But I also enjoy the challenge—and the kick—of getting it right the first time.

Fifty minutes fly by. John breaks for ten to let us rest our chops. Susan, my flute section mate, walks with me to the water fountain. One circuit around the school has become our intermission ritual. Susan waits, holding my flute for me, while I pop into the ladies' room, where Deb and I compare notes on the music so far. As Susan and I complete our circuit, we exchange friendly hellos with our baritone horn player, Walter. It took me a season before I learned his last name, and another season to confirm what I suspected: Walter MacLean is the pediatric allergist who told my mother—so many years and so many towns ago—to start me on a wind instrument.

An hour later I am swabbing out my flute, packing up my instrument. I walk Bob to his car. He once told me he feels great after every rehearsal. "It's like doing two hours of yoga," he said. Like yoga, playing a wind instrument asks us to regulate and control our breathing. And like yoga, music asks us to focus. In most of our rehearsals, there are times when I think of other things—times when John is asking the lower brass or the trumpets to play and replay a line and my mind drifts away from the music and back to the demands of the day or the worries of tomorrow. But reading well requires that you give your undivided attention to the music on your stand. It's a lot like a concert, but with none of the pressure.

"We sounded pretty good in May," Bob says as he opens his car door. Bob's wife videotapes every concert, and he makes a point to watch the tape and listen carefully to every performance. "I was pretty pleased."

"You played a great concert," I affirm.

"The tone's there. That's what matters to me. The fingers aren't what they used to be, but as long as I still have that tone, I'll keep playing."

"You have a beautiful sound. You'd better keep playing. Your first clarinet colleagues are all good players, but you have something—fullness—and a maturity they just can't match."

"At my age, I would hope I have maturity," Bob says with a laugh. "See you next week!"

I look forward to seeing Bob next week, and for weeks and years to come. I've always appreciated his playing, but when I first joined the band, Bob intimidated me. I knew he'd been playing forever, that he took rehearsals seriously, and I could see his occasional impatience with some members of our group. Clearly, he had high standards and I had better live up to them if I wanted his respect. Through seasons of playing together, our musical relationship was formed, and I discovered Bob was not so scary. He had a sense of humor—a sometimes wicked sense of humor at that. The band was arranged a little differently then, so Bob sat right behind me. As our musical relationship deepened, I came to feel that Bob was watching my back. I came to rely on his certainty when I felt less secure.

It was a few years later, during pre-op tests for his planned back surgery, that doctors discovered Bob's cancer. He showed up for rehearsals almost every week while he was undergoing treatment.

"It's great that you're here."

"I'd rather be here than not," he said.

That was the season he told me, "I'm relying on you to carry me through that passage." It was series of rapid sixteenth notes we shared.

For just a few months, our roles reversed. I was happy to be able to support Bob, to give him back some of the musical security he'd so graciously afforded me.

The next year we changed concert venues and John rearranged the band. I still sit to John's left on the far end of the front row, but Bob now sits second-row center. At first I hated this new arrangement, for it makes it harder for Bob and me to hear each other. But over time it's worked out fine. Bob has returned to full-strength, and I've found my own strength through Bob's temporary reliance on me. We're equal partners who look to each other for support. And the new seating arrangement has another advantage: Bob and I can see each other now. We share secret smiles after a passage well played, and we roll our eyes at each other when that new trumpet player decides to warm up with deafening, stratospheric high notes again.

I'm still thinking about Bob as I pull into my driveway. I think about my grandmother. I think about my mother. "Don't get old, Katie."

I consider there are various ways to get old. I vote for Bob's way. Showing up every week to play music, come hell or high water, and vowing to keep playing until I lose my tone.

Chapter Eight

Forgetting

"Try to imagine what it would be like to wake up in the morning without your memory."

Suzanne gives me a moment to conjure up my bedroom—the way the morning light peeks through the blinds, the weight of the covers on me as I wake—where I'm warm, and most likely needing to pee. As I place Bix—purring—next to me in my imaginary morning, I stumble on the paradox: in the act of imagining the loss of my memory, I am using my unlost memory like crazy. That's Suzanne's point. We depend on our memories to guide us through every moment of every day. We spend our infanthood learning the basics—how to suck and swallow, how to chew, how to walk, how to recognize hunger or pain, and how to communicate our needs to others. What we learn—and what we remember—gains sophistication, subtlety, as we progress from infant to toddler to child to young adult.

"From everything you've told me, your mother still remembers the basic things to do when she wakes up in the morning. But there may be some parts of the sequence missing. She may have forgotten that part of her routine is showering. Or eating breakfast. Or it may be that she just can't remember or manage the sequence of steps we follow to take a shower or make breakfast. You and I don't think about our morning routines—we just do them—but every day, we rely on a process of remembering and following a sequence of steps."

Suzanne is an elder-care consultant. She has come to me through a circuitous route that began with my sister-in-law, Martha, an RN and elder-care advocate in northern Maine. Martha, who is also working on her doctorate in history, has been helping me long-distance. "We need to find you someone closer," she told me when we last spoke. Before I could check out the online list she sent me, my hairdresser gave me a brochure from a client who specialized in health care advocacy. Two phone calls and an e-mail later, I was put me in touch with Suzanne.

Now she is sitting at my dining room table, exuding calm and caring. Suzanne has strong features, wide cheekbones, dark brown eyes, and pale blonde, wavy hair that brushes her shoulders. She seems put together in a way that makes me slightly self-conscious of my jeans and sweater. I find that as she speaks, Suzanne's voice—slightly nasal and with minimal inflections—relaxes me. She seems both efficient and empathic—a rare and winning combination.

I've told Suzanne that I have been worried about my mother's nutrition, and her words are confirming my worst fears: my mother has most likely forgotten not only how to prepare food but also when she needs to eat. As for the showering in the morning, well, that hasn't been a part of my mother's routine for some time. I've wondered whether her smoking has so blunted her sense of smell that she doesn't realize just how ripe she is. And I've been chalking up the reluctance to shower to her fear of falling, or to the trouble she has climbing over the wall of the tub, or even to the way her hip makes it difficult to stay balanced in a standing position. I've been looking into shower chairs, handrails, and other assistive devices with which we might retrofit her tub. In the meantime, I have been inviting her over to my house for a once-a-week dinner, shower, and sleepover.

I crank up the heat, make sure the water is running hot, and help her into the tub. She's wrapped in a towel at this point, which she hands to me only after she instructs me not to look. Obedient, I reach in for the towel, then stand on the other side of the curtain in case she feels unsteady. I hand her a facecloth, remind her to use soap, remind her to scrub her underarms.

When she says she's done, I reach in again to turn off the water. Then I hand her back the towel.

"Don't look at me. I'm naked!" she says.

"Not looking, just providing the linens," I assure her, doing my best to give her privacy and dignity in this operation. I have warm clothes ready for her as soon as she steps out of the tub—I'd put them in the dryer just before I turned on the water. She's always cold, and often she uses this as her excuse for not showering.

"I'll just shower in the morning at home," she'll say to me, and even though I know this will never happen, I'm still not sure whether she is just trying to shut me up or whether she actually believes, in that moment, that she will shower the next morning.

On the nights when I can't coax her into the shower—and there have been more of them recently as the weather gets colder—I do my best to accomplish some sort of cleanup. Because I do my mother's laundry now, I always have clean clothes here for her. And I bought her some teddy bear pajamas to tempt her out of her day clothes and into some nightclothes.

"I'm fine as I am," she says. "I'm too cold to take any clothes off!"

I've tried different techniques to persuade my mother to give up her always-smelly clothes and to put on some pj's, but on some nights I realize I can't win. She will crawl under the covers of the pullout bed and tell me she doesn't know how I can stand to live in such a cold house.

On the mornings when she wakes up in her clothes, I know better than to suggest a morning shower. "Are you kidding me? Wet hair on a day like this?"

"Mom, you need a sponge bath." The terminology dates back to my grandmother, and maybe for this reason, my mother is marginally less resistant to the concept.

"Oh, I'll do that when I get home."

"No, Mom. I need to get those dirty clothes off you and into the laundry. Plus, you are a little stinky." This is the phrase she finds least insulting, and sometimes the idea of being a little stinky even makes her laugh.

"That's just my natural fragrant aroma. I smell like violets," she says, grinning.

"Stinky violets. Let's get you washed up and changed so we can go out to lunch."

"The ladies who lunch," my mother says.

"Exactly, and they don't let stinky ladies to lunch."

She giggles and allows me to lead her to the bathroom. I help her take off her top, unbuckle her sad little threadbare bra. I have a warm, soapy washcloth ready. I work on her back, her arms, her underarms.

"I need your slacks and panties to add to the load I'm going to put into the laundry."

"Okay, but I don't want you to see me naked!"

"I'll turn around and you can just hand them to me." I give her another warm, soapy washcloth and tell her she needs to wash the rest of her body herself. I stay long enough to listen, to hear the wetness of the cloth hit skin, and then I leave her, but not before she says, "I'm freezing, Katie! Why do you keep your house so goddamn cold?"

∽

"The inability to keep up with personal hygiene is one of the classic signs of Alzheimer's," Suzanne tells me, "and family members are often most bothered by this particular change in behavior."

Several months ago—it was in the summertime, when she was willing to take off the sneakers that she would wear to bed if I let her—my mother complained about not being able to see her foot doctor.

I reassured her I was working on the health insurance issue. "But if you need to see him now, maybe we should check to see how much he costs without insurance," I added.

"Oh, he's too much money, even with insurance! A hundred and fifty dollars just to cut my toenails!"

"I'm sure he does more than cut your toenails."

"Oh, he shaves that thing on the bottom of my foot, but what I really need is a pedicure."

For a couple of years now, I've been helping my mother with her fingernails. The arthritis in her hands makes it impossible for her to squeeze the clipper, but she is fine with an emery board. I clip; she files; then we scrub her fingernails, take off all the old polish, and apply new. It's a job we usually do seated at my kitchen island. When she first asked for my help, I was a little thrown. I keep my fingernails short—better for flute playing and for writing on a computer keyboard—and my mother's long nails frighten me just a bit. Perhaps we'd be better off making an appointment at a nail salon? No, my mother seemed to want my help with her manicure.

I don't exactly enjoy clipping my mother's fingernails, but there is something about holding her fingertips in my hands that feels special, almost precious.

Maybe that's why I offered to do her toenails.

"I just can't reach my own toes anymore."

If there had been a hint of apology or defensiveness in my mother's tone, I might have been prepared for what I saw when she took off her sneakers. But she was matter-of-fact, and I thought it best to hold that tone as I caught my first glance of her overgrown toenails, inches too long, curving around her toes.

How long, I wondered, *has it been since her nails were clipped? How painful must this be?*

My mother has always had mobility issues—she was diagnosed with degenerative arthritis of the spine when she was in her thirties—and her visits to the foot doctor, she has told me, are necessary because there is a bone in her foot that faces the wrong way, causing a bunion and calluses to form. But as I stared at her feet, I wondered how much of her difficulty with balance and movement might have been a result of her inability to cut her own toenails.

"Let's begin with a good washing," I suggested.

I had the washcloth—warm, soapy—ready. We were in her living room. She was seated on the loveseat with the New England lighthouse upholstery. I was seated at her feet. I pushed her ancient sneakers and socks away from me to eliminate some of the unpleasant odor, and I began.

I channeled some other version of myself, detached, neutral. But I felt emotionally devastated. In baring her feet to me, my mother seemed to be confirming my worst fears. My mind and my heart were racing, but my hands moved in comforting motions and my face revealed, I am pretty sure, nothing to my mother. My poor, poor mother.

I focused on the process: wash, towel dry, apply moisturizer.

Why did they leave out this part of "Rip Van Winkle"? How

long were Sleeping Beauty's nails when she was awakened with a kiss?

"Your nails are kind of long," I said, Mistress of Understatement. "This may take a while. I'm going to wrap one foot up so you don't get cold while I work on the other."

"Whatever you think." My mother, relaxing into her mini foot spa, was agreeable.

I considered the possibility that this situation might require professional intervention. I was afraid her nails might not fit under my clipper or that they might be too hard and resist cutting. I was worried that I might hurt my mother. But I forged ahead, making several passes on each toenail, and in about twenty minutes my mother's feet were in good shape. I suggested another quick footbath, applied more moisturizer, and pulled clean socks onto my mother's feet.

"How much do you charge for that?" she asked me.

∽

I don't share the foot story with Suzanne. It seems too personal. But it's another example of my not knowing what to think. Were my mother's unkempt toenails a function of her inability to reach her toes, or her inability to ask for help, or her inability to remember that she needs to do something about her toenails? And her attachment to those rotting sneakers—I've bought her two new pairs, one white, one black, but she will not give up the pair with the floppy sole and the growing hole on the side of her big toe. She claims the new white sneakers aren't as comfortable. "And the black ones just look like death."

I feel locked in this constant process of evaluation. How much of my mother's behavior is long-standing? How much is new? How much is harmless eccentricity? How much stems from physical incapacity? How much from diminished mental capacity? For a while now, I've understood that my mother is experiencing some form of memory loss, but I have been careful not to label it. Not only out of fear, but also out of some misguided notion of respect.

Now Suzanne is using the term *Alzheimer's*, and despite everything I have read, everything I have observed about my mother, I'm having trouble hearing that word.

"Is it true that a definitive diagnosis of Alzheimer's is impossible until the point of autopsy?" I ask Suzanne.

"It's technically true you can't see Alzheimer's in a living brain, the way you could see a broken bone or a tumor. But we know enough about the disease and the way it progresses to be able to diagnose it on the basis of changes in behavior, and a CT scan tells us something about the physical state of the brain."

"So I need to get her to a doctor and get these tests ordered."

"Yes, but what is more important now is making sure your mother is safe. If she is going to stay in her house, you need to notify the Yarmouth police—"

"The police? Why the police?"

"In case something happens or she wanders or gets in an accident."

"What you're really saying is that you don't believe she is safe to live alone."

"Again, I haven't met your mother yet—but from what you've told me, no. In circumstances like this, the best situation is usually assisted living. It's what I would recommend here—if you can find a way to pay for it. And sooner is better. It will only get harder to move her out of her house. She's expressed willingness to move, and I'd advise you to take advantage of that before she changes her mind."

〜

I know from the reading I've already done that forgetting, in an Alzheimer's patient, follows the reverse path of learning and remembering. First we forget the most recent things we've learned—what we had for lunch, perhaps—and then we forget how to make lunch. Next we forget we need to eat lunch. Ultimately, we will forget *how* to eat lunch. In the end, we will forget the first things we learned in this life: how to suck and how to swallow.

No one dies of Alzheimer's. The disease does not ravage the body the way a terminal cancer does. Alzheimer's patients simply forget how to stay alive.

Without round-the-clock supervision, a late-stage patient could choke to death. Without a feeding tube, she could starve. It's a horrible, horrible outcome, and one I hope my mother will not experience. Yet I understand this is a possible future for my mother, for me.

When I share what I know—and what I fear—about this disease, Suzanne tells me that Alzheimer's is a long-lived, slow-moving illness. "The difference between Alzheimer's and other forms of dementia is that Alzheimer's is progressive and predictable."

She explains that in the medical profession, there is some dispute in the staging of the disease process but general agreement that the disease progresses in identifiable phases. "I prefer to think of four stages. We can determine, through various tests, which stage your mother is in, and then we will have a better sense of what the future might look like. My guess, based on how you have described her, is early stage two. Now each stage can last from three to seven years—"

"Seven years?" A quick calculation: if it took seven years

to reach this point, and my mother takes seven years to pass through each stage—we could be in this for twenty-one more years. My mother will be nearing ninety, and I will be sixty-six and possibly four years into my own process of forgetting.

"Don't worry about that right now," Suzanne says, and I wonder whether she is reading my mind. "It's easy to miss the early signs, especially if the patient lives alone. And I suspect some part of your mother's dementia is what we call vascular dementia—that means the blood supply to the brain is inadequate. It's common with smokers. Vascular dementia is less predicable, because there is no telling exactly what part of the brain will be affected by the diminished blood supply. My guess is your mother has a combination."

Suzanne encourages me to call my mother's doctor and to visit some assisted living facilities. She loads me up with handouts and asks me to send back a survey form to Alzheimer's Services of Cape Cod. Her complimentary home visit is covered by a grant to provide assistance and support to caregivers. I feel like I should not only fill out the survey but also write them a thank-you note. The two hours I have spent with Suzanne have flown by. I've learned a lot, but even more, I've been comforted by sitting with someone who has no fear or judgment around memory loss. Suzanne is compassionate and yet also matter-of-fact. She doesn't shrink from the bitter realities, but her focus is to keep the patient safe and the caregivers sane. We have shared goals.

"Can I hire you?" I ask her as she is gathering her stuff to leave.

She suggests we talk after I visit Sunrise and Pocasset—two assisted living facilities. "The grant covers a little more time, so let's do a follow-up call after you have more information."

My question was impulsive, and I'm grateful for her measured answer. It's clear to me that I need Suzanne on my team. What's not clear is how I can afford her time.

"You have a beautiful home," she says just before she leaves.

"Thanks. And thanks so much for your time and expertise."

"You'll be fine," she says with surprising conviction. She smiles. "Talk to you soon. Remember," she adds, "you never have to be alone in this."

I nod and smile, but the truth is, as I watch Suzanne get into her car, I feel alone. Alone and a little aggrieved. Scared out of my mind and overwhelmed.

I close the door. *Alzheimer's.* God, I hate that word.

Chapter Nine

So Sue Me

"I'd like to sue my daughter," my mother says to the attorney. "Is that something you can handle for me?"

"Mom—ahh—I don't think he's that kind of lawyer." I smile, hoping the attorney and witnesses we have gathered will assume my mother is kidding.

In fact, she has been threatening to sue since she slipped off the stool in my kitchen. I was at the sink across the counter, and I saw her take the fall, but I can't say for sure what happened. She moved from sitting to almost standing before she appeared to crumple to the floor. My friend Bruce, who was occupying the other counter stool, reached for her. But she went down too fast.

"Mom, are you okay?" I was on my knees next to her.

"My hip, goddamn it."

"What about your back?"

"My back is fine, but my fanny is killing me. Why are your floors so damn slippery? I'm going to sue you!"

"You probably bruised your tailbone, Mom. You didn't hit your head, did you?"

"No, goddamn it! I landed on my fanny. Ouch!"

"You'll be sore for a few days, but I don't think you've broken anything. How about some ice?"

"Ice! Your house is already too goddamn cold!" She sat down on the loveseat in the living room. "My fanny hurts like hell! Ouch! I'm going to sue you!"

"Well, there's not much you'd get out of a lawsuit, Mom. Kind of like blood from a stone?"

A smile, and then a shift of position. "Ow! My fanny hurts! I'm going to sue you, Kathleen."

My mother has threatened legal action every time she notices that her butt hurts. As best as I can figure, she forgets about the injury until she sits on her tailbone a certain way, and then— bam—she remembers she fell, determines my slippery floors are to blame, and feels the impulse to sue me all over again. This has been happening, on average, about twenty times a day for the past six days. It's getting on my nerves.

If I were less annoyed by her repeated threats to sue me, I might find it more interesting that she has reinvented the story of her fall. She begins to tell the attorney that she was walking down the hallway when she fell. The cause? Not her hip. Not her balance issues. My slippery wood floors. She seems to have forgotten falling off the stool, but she is clinging to this new version of events, which, I have to admit, does more to support her claim. My kitchen floor is covered in nineteen-year-old linoleum with no shine left in it. Slippery, it is not.

The attorney to whom she relates her tale of household injustice is, thank God, a man. A tall man who is wearing a suit. "Well, Anne, I am that kind of attorney too. But what do you say we get these documents in order before we discuss your lawsuit against your daughter?" My mother is satisfied and charmed. When he chuckles, she does too. On the whole, and despite her own impressive career, my mother prefers men, especially in positions of authority, and especially tall men, who remind her of my father.

We're meeting at my accountant's office. Kathey has been

doing my taxes forever—since she was a one-woman show sharing her crowded quarters with a computer business run by the man who is now her ex. These days she has nicely appointed offices, several folks working for her, and a new husband. She also looks about ten years younger than she did when I first met her, which means she has reversed her aging process by about twice that many years. I'm pretty sure her secret is happiness.

Kathey's office is in Osterville, a wealthy little village on Cape Cod, and most of her clients have what might be genteelly called "resources." The elder-law attorney she recommended was from a high-priced law firm outside Boston—no doubt the sort of prestigious contact most of her clients would prefer. When I'd met with him a few months ago, he was kind and helpful. He made several recommendations, some more expensive to carry out than others and some just not necessary for folks of our limited means. I've decided to stick with the bargain package: power of attorney, health care proxy, and a revision of my mother's will. At some point she made changes in her own handwriting to the original document.

As the attorney begins passing out the paperwork, Kathey tells my mother how great it is to see her. Kathey's office manager, Katherine, compliments my mother on the Celtic cross she is wearing around her neck.

"I bought it in Ireland," my mother declares.

I am grateful my mother has been distracted from the pain in her tailbone. When Katherine asks about the trip to Ireland, my mother says she has been several times and that she studied one summer at Trinity College in Dublin. What comes next surprises me.

"The people in Dublin are lovely," my mother says. "So friendly and generous—not like the people in Paris, which is where my daughter prefers to travel."

"Oh, have you been to Paris too?" Kathey asks.

I might have asked the same question myself. If my mother has seen Paris, this is the first I've ever heard of it.

"I only spent a day there. But that was enough! We took the train from Paris to London and then flew over to Ireland."

"Oh, you took the Chunnel train? How was that?" asks Katherine.

"Fine, but the people in Paris—they were so rude! I wouldn't want to spend any time in that city! But my daughter—*she* loves it there."

My mother is trying to get a rise out of me. She wants me to defend Paris, my adopted city and the setting of a novel I finished writing this fall. The digs about Paris, the threats to sue—they spring from the same well of anger. My mother isn't happy to be at the attorney's today; she doesn't like the way I am "controlling" her life. She's mad at me, and she wants me to be mad back.

I shrug and smile, not only to keep the peace but because I don't know whether my mother has been to Paris. *Was the Chunnel finished in time for her last trip to Ireland? Why would anyone go through Paris to get to London to get to Dublin? And after all my trips to Paris, why would she mention this to me for the first time now? But would she just make up a day in Paris?*

My mother has invented the slippery floor story, and in recent months she has reengineered several other truths to suit her purposes. She swore, for example, that she dropped her car keys when she was getting out of her car in the dark. She called me to come root around in the dirt under the car. No keys were found in the vicinity. Yet she would not budge from the story she had come to believe was true: she had dropped the keys, in the dark, in the rain, and they were somewhere under the car. "I just hope someone hasn't stolen them."

After I persuaded her that we should look inside the house,

I found the keys hiding between the cushions of her living room loveseat.

The lost and found keys, the kitchen turned hallway, and now this Paris story: I am coming to understand that when my mother forgets something—but not everything—about a situation, she becomes creative. She fashions a story that might be true, and then she clings to her reinvention. What's remarkable is that she is able to hold on to the new mythology. Assert, repeat, repeat, repeat. And me? Unless I am a witness to the original truth—like the upset in my kitchen—I have no idea where the line between fact and fiction is drawn. Has my mother been to Paris? Has she taken the Chunnel train? It seems so unlikely—but my mother, the drama coach, is still a great actress and a persuasive speaker. Is her Celtic cross from a little shop in Dublin? I'm not sure. Maybe. Part of me feels like a traitor for doubting her. I check back into the conversation and hear my mother claiming the Irish knit sweater she is wearing today as a souvenir from the Irish countryside. *Ireland?* Try T. J. Maxx.

We move through the meeting. When my mother complains I am taking over her life, the lawyer explains that the power of attorney just gives me copilot status and that the health care proxy only comes into play if she is unable to make a medical decision herself.

"Yes, yes. I understand," my mother says, waving away further discussion with her fly-swatting voice. She signs each document, and Kathey and Katherine sign as witnesses. Their signatures and the attorney's oversight of these transactions affirm that my mother is of sound mind. On the way home, I can't shake the feeling that we got those papers signed just in the nick of time.

∽

We return to my house and to Bruce, a friend for more than twenty years, a bookseller who is presently between bookstores. His between-jobs status has allowed him the flexibility to extend what is usually a two-day holiday visit, and I've been taking advantage of his presence to check out the assisted living facilities that Suzanne has recommended. My mother has been with me now for ten days, and I don't feel comfortable leaving her in the house alone. I worry about the many small things she could forget—to turn off the teakettle, to make sure Bix stays inside when she steps outside for a smoke. And since the fall from the stool, I worry about her stability moving from room to room.

These ten days have opened my eyes. The forgetting that my mother is able to mask with her still-superior verbal skills reveals itself in proximity. Every day I see that what Suzanne has told me is true: my mother has trouble moving through her day. She has forgotten any number of usual sequences. And her conversational repetition—which I had been thinking could be a side effect of her isolation—is even worse in company. She isn't only repeating stories but repeating questions, and just moments after she has received her answer.

My own mechanisms of denial and hopefulness have been swept aside too. I see now that it is unsafe for my mother to live alone. Not in a little house or a nearby condo or apartment—even for the short term. And my fantasies of the perfect shared domicile—fading for a while—have been entirely erased in the span of less than two weeks. I see that, on my own, I cannot provide the care that she needs. Suzanne—and my uncle Jack, who has been pushing assisted living for some time—are right. The interim solutions I'd imagined are not solutions at all.

Perhaps because my mother senses that I am seeing her vulnerabilities, she has been less inclined, these past several days, to tamp down her anger—all of it directed squarely at me. It's been tough to take, and a couple of days ago I lost it.

"Do you really think I am enjoying this?" I asked her, after she'd accused me of trying to run—and ruin—her life for the umpteenth time. "Do you think I want you in my house, criticizing my every move, complaining about everything? Do you think your nastiness makes me *want* to help you? Jesus, Mom. You are in trouble and I'm doing what a daughter is *supposed* to do. It would be nice if you could appreciate that, but God knows that would be asking *way* too much of you. You've never noticed anything I've done—*ever*."

"Don't kid yourself. You've always been a selfish bitch."

"They say the apple doesn't fall far from the tree."

I remember leaving the room—the living room—and hoping in that moment that my mother wasn't really my tree, that I was not her apple, or that at least I had been picked when ripened and carted far, far away. But before I was halfway down the hall, I felt awful about our angry exchange, about losing my temper. I'd known from the start of this journey into my mother's late-life business that I needed to let go of all the longstanding mother-daughter issues between us, that I needed to give my mother the understanding and goodwill that I would extend to any human being in need of my help and protection. I gave myself a good reprimand, and then I decided I could give myself the benefit of human kindness too. The only way I'll get through this, I realized, is to go a little easy on myself.

"Care for the caregiver," Suzanne said to me when we met last week. But I really didn't take it in. After all, I am not usually with my mother 24/7. If she moves into assisted living, I will see her once or twice a week. I won't be bathing her or dressing her or seeing that she gets her meals every day. Am I a caregiver? I care for my mother, about my mother, and about every little thing that makes a difference in her life. I *give care*. Awkward usage, my English teacher mom would have told me a few years back, but I'm going with it. I am giving care, and thus I must take care too.

"She's just so ceaseless," Bruce had said to me earlier in the week. "I don't know where you find the patience. And some of the things she says about you when you're gone—it takes all I have in me not to give her a good talking-to, to tell her she ought to be happy she has a daughter who cares about her—especially with the way she acts toward you."

"You're seeing her at her worst," I told Bruce. "Truly, we have had some okay moments. Not so many lately. She's mad a lot now. But really, can you blame her?"

There was a pause, perhaps while Bruce was weighing blame, before he said "Bless you" and announced he was going for a walk.

After my outburst, I didn't feel deserving of any blessing. And clearly I had no patience. But in my newfound determination to go easier on myself, I saw a simple solution: an apology. It would make us both feel better.

My mother was still seated in the same chair in the living room. She looked up from her reading and smiled at me. Perhaps twenty minutes after calling me a selfish bitch, she had already forgotten the harsh words between us. Not in the forgive-and-forget way of forgetting. She had no recollection of our argument. None. And no anger or obvious resentment, not in that moment.

"How about a cup of coffee, Katie? And maybe something sweet? Some of that cake you made would be so nice."

I moved into the kitchen to put on the kettle, and I realized that my mother's forgetting, while letting me off the hook this time, meant I was absolutely, for sure, on the hook. Forevermore.

Chapter Ten

Sundown at Sunrise

I have discovered, in these past three weeks, that my mother is a compulsive hummer. She hums the same sequence of notes— the beginning, or perhaps the middle, of a tune I do not recognize. She pauses for a moment before she begins again. Hum, pause, repeat. Pause, hum, pause. Repeat, pause, hum. It makes me crazy. The melody never progresses. There is no line, no phrase, no resolution. She hums, not occasionally, but pretty much all the time.

The humming, the threats to sue, the cycles of repetition that have become routine: I can see no way for my mother to live with me unless I give up working altogether. Home, for me, is also workplace, and the work I do requires focus, concentration, and a measure of silence. My mother is silent only when she sleeps. That's if you don't count the snoring—which I don't. I can work through the rhythmic snuffles of sleep time. But I cannot work through the humming. It creates static in my brain; it's like I am between radio stations and I can't tune in the one I want to hear because I can't tune out the adjacent station.

I am starting to understand that Suzanne is right. Assisted living is, most likely, the best possible scenario for my mother— and for me. As I pull into Sunrise of Plymouth, I hope this might be somewhere my mother could be happy. Including Sunrise, I've visited four assisted living facilities, winnowed down from the many more I have checked out by phone or online. One was well priced, well situated, and with a nice feeling—but it was two hours away from me. Another, just a few miles from my home, was super expensive and the food was awful. The best fit so far was on the Cape, in a lovely wooded setting, with a roomy, subsidized apartment. My mother met the income standards, but was disqualified by the equity in her home. Sunrise is part of a chain of facilities offering assisted living as well as more intensive Alzheimer's care. Suzanne had suggested I check this one out.

My first visit to Sunrise of Plymouth coincides with afternoon snack time. Most of the residents are in the lobby, seated at café tables, drinking coffee and eating freshly baked chocolate chip cookies. As I check in with the receptionist, I wonder if they plan introductory visits for this time of day. Taking in the sights and sounds of sociability, I consider that if it is a ploy, it's working.

Noreen, the community representative, comes to the desk to meet me. She's forty-something, with long blonde hair and a bright smile. She shows me around, explaining how the building is divided into T- and L-shaped wings called "cottages," each housing fifteen to twenty residents. The cottages are named after trees. She mentions Elm, Aspen, Oak. "Let's look at Aspen first. I have a studio and a one-bedroom available there. The other opening is in Elm, on the second floor."

Our first stop is the dining room for the Aspen cottage. The afternoon sunlight is streaming into a room decorated in yellow, blue, and white. There are six wooden tables, each with four chairs. I notice the chair cushions and think of my mother's bony bum. She's forever complaining about the hardness of chairs, stools, benches.

"I know some places have large central dining, but we find this setup makes mealtimes friendlier and less overwhelming for our residents," Noreen says. We cross the hallway to look at the studio that is available on this floor. It's small, to be sure, but laid out in such a way that it doesn't feel cramped. I like the fact that it is near the kitchen—maybe my mother will eat more regularly—and close to the lobby and the front doors.

I follow Noreen down a long corridor to the living room. It is equipped with a gas fireplace surrounded by built-in bookcases (with a lousy book selection), a large-screen TV, several wing chairs, a couch, and a table with four chairs around it. "The ladies in Aspen like to play cards at night. And sometimes Scrabble." Noreen smiles. I know my mother hates card games, but she might be talked into Scrabble.

"We host family parties in these living rooms. You just need to book ahead. We can even cater it for you."

I find myself picturing my mother's family coming to Sunrise for a holiday party. I don't know if it is the layout, the warm colors on the walls, the gathering in the lobby, or my helpful tour guide stopping to greet every resident by name, but I feel like my mother just might be able to live here, be safe, and enjoy herself.

Noreen shows me the larger apartment. Lovely, with a woodland view, but beyond our means.

"We have one apartment like this in every cottage, and they are great for couples. Most of our residents live in studios. We like to encourage folks to get out of their rooms and socialize. That doesn't happen if everybody has a big apartment of their own."

We go upstairs to see the studio in the Elm cottage. It has an ocean view in the wintertime, but it would require my mother to go up and down stairs or take an elevator. She isn't fond of either activity.

Back in Noreen's office, I inform her that my mother is a smoker.

"Of course there is no smoking in the building, but we have covered areas for smoking outside, and we have a buzzer system in case your mom goes out for a smoke after seven o'clock, when we lock the front doors. I'd recommend you take that room on the first floor. It will be easier for her to get out. There's a pretty lively group in the Aspen cottage. I believe two of the ladies smoke, so she'll have company. Your mother will be one of our younger residents, so I think she'd be happier with a group that is more active. There's another retired teacher in Aspen—Geri. I think your mother will fit in nicely."

Noreen seems to understand that I worry about my mother making friends, pretty much the same way a parent would worry about her child making friends in a new school—a boarding school, in this case. And like Suzanne, Noreen is sympathetic yet matter-of-fact about my mother's deteriorating mental faculties—calm and unafraid to use the word *Alzheimer's*.

"Almost everybody in this building has some memory loss. That's why we have Suzanne come in once a week to provide staff training. Most of the residents are like your mother—still able to function pretty well, but in need of a little assistance— regular meals, help with a shower once a week, that sort of thing. In the Alzheimer's cottages, we provide a higher level of care and there are fewer residents. Otherwise they operate just about the same way, and they look the same—except they are secured. Would you like to see them?"

I would. One of the reasons Suzanne has suggested Sunrise is that they have an Alzheimer's component in the same build-ing. In a best-case scenario, my mother can just move down the hall when she needs more assistance and support.

We go back upstairs, this time heading away from the Elm

cottage. Noreen uses a security code to unlock a set of auto-matic double doors, and we are in.

In my mother's possible future.

Yes, I do want to see, but I am afraid to look.

We pass the dining room—cheerful and casual, like the dining rooms in the unsecured cottages. Most of the residents' doors are open, and as we walk down the corridor, I can see the beds are made and the rooms look homey. The residents—all women on this floor—are in the living room.

Noreen introduces me. They nod at her, smile, and say hello to me. "How are you doing today?" Noreen asks the room at large. She receives a few positive replies and some more smiles.

My guess is that most of these women spend their days in small, self-contained worlds. Aside from two who seem to be sharing some sort of task that involves yarn, these residents seem unlikely to interact without prompting. Their social skills are more like reflexes—present, but only evident when acti-vated with a direct question.

"I think Barbara has some games for you," Noreen says. Another staff member has appeared with a plastic tote—filled, evidently, with suitable activities. "I'll leave you to it." The resi-dents' attention has already focused on Barbara, leaving me free of social convention. I'm not sure I could have managed *It was nice meeting you.* The doors lock behind us automatically. Ad-vancing Alzheimer's patients are likely to wander, to get lost. I understand that the security is necessary. But I feel relieved my mother won't be living in a locked unit—not yet.

Downstairs, the second secured cottage looks and feels much like the first. There is a weird feeling of absence, even though all residents are present and accounted for—and gath-ered, once again, in the comfy living room.

"Cats," I say before Noreen has a chance to introduce me.

"Yes. Aren't they great? We allow small pets in all the cottages, but we require that the residents or their families care for them—walking, litter box, that sort of thing."

My mother's cat will not be making the trip to Sunrise. Emily disappeared just a few weeks ago. I posted signs, made circuits of my mother's neighborhood, knocked on doors, asked folks to check their garages and sheds. She never turned up. I'm hoping that Emily—a former feral with a knack for survival—has relocated to a smoke-free home where she is well fed and well loved.

"These two came over from Elm with one of the women who is here now," Noreen is saying. "With Nancy, I think. Nancy, are these your cats?" One of the women, dressed impeccably but until that moment looking vacant, comes to attention. She nods.

"They're beautiful," I say, squatting down to pat the spotted tiger as the Siamese swishes by to investigate.

Nancy smiles, nods at me. "My cats."

The others in the room seem pleased with the cats too. The cats are pleased in turn. They begin to make the rounds, catching pats and smiles from the ladies in the circle.

Before we leave, a man in a wheelchair grabs Noreen's arm.

"There's been a mistake. I need you to call my daughter. I don't belong here. All these people are crazy. Look at them! I'm not crazy. I don't belong here. I need you to call my daughter."

"I can't call your daughter," Noreen told him, "but I'll make sure to give the message to the nurse."

"There's been a mistake," he says again. "I need you to call my daughter." He repeats himself word for word.

Noreen does not vary her response.

He seems calmer for a moment before he begins again: "There's been a mistake."

Is he becoming agitated with the repetitions—or am I? I've learned from my interactions with my mother that individuals with memory loss do not repeat themselves for the reasons the rest of us do. This gentleman isn't worried that we didn't hear him, or frustrated that his message isn't getting across, or annoyed that we haven't already acted on his request. He has simply forgotten that he's already told his story to Noreen. As we head to the doorway, he follows us in his wheelchair.

"There's been a mistake—" The fifth repetition in four minutes.

"I know." Noreen says to him, as she looks straight at him. "I'll take care of it."

~

"Have you heard of sundowning?" Dave asks me. He's Noreen's colleague, and he was back in the office when we returned.

I nod. It's a not uncommon but mostly unexplained phenomenon in Alzheimer's patients: they seem to go downhill as the day turns to night. Their repetitive cycle amps up. They can get agitated. They seem to slide into a deeper stage of dementia, if only for an hour. Suzanne told me patients will often ask—repeatedly—to go home, even if they are living at home.

When I nod, Dave says, "I'm pretty sure that's what is going on with Clark—the man you just met. He's new to us, though, so we need to be sure he is in the right place. Sometimes people think their family members need more support than they really do."

I can see how that could happen. Living with my mother for the past few weeks, I have begun to wonder whether she needs more care than the basic level most assisted living facilities offer. But now that I have met the residents behind those locked doors, I understand that my mother, while absolutely in need of assistance, is not in need of round-the-clock security. She may not be showering on any regular basis, and she may be forgetting to eat. She may be cycling and recycling through the same conversations with me, and she may need an arm to lean on when she is going up or down stairs. But she is still socially adept—so much so that she tricked me into believing she was okay for a long, long time. I'm not sure whether that gentleman's daughter has made a mistake or he actually is in the right place, but I am relieved that my mother will be eating her chocolate chip cookies in the main lobby.

Still, I'm glad I visited the Alzheimer's cottages. They weren't awful. With the exception of the man in the wheelchair, the residents didn't seem to be unhappy. They were safe, cared for, and perhaps, in some way that was not visible to me, content in each others' company. I don't want to envision my mother in that silent circle of women—at least not for a long time—but if she were there . . . well, I think it would be a lot better than any number of other places she could be.

On my way back to the Cape, I time the ride: forty minutes door to door without traffic—manageable, as long as I plan my travel for off-peak hours during the tourist season. I'm feeling good about Sunrise. I can picture my mother, coffee and cookie, chatting with the friends she would make. Friends she would never make living on her own—or with me. A woman named Marilyn had offered to show me her room and promised me that she would make sure my mother felt right at home. "Does she play cards?" she asked. Before I could answer that one, she asked, "Does she like to shop?" and began to show me some of the bargains she'd found at a nearby thrift shop. "The bus takes us there. Oh, don't you worry. We'll have fun, your mother and me."

❧

As soon as I get home, I call to check on my mother. At her insistence, she's back in her house—at least until the next snowstorm.

"How much?" my mother asks, after I tell her about my trip to Sunrise.

"I think we can afford it," I say, not answering her question.

"Well, not until the house sells—and that will be the spring at the earliest."

If someone gave me a dollar for every time that my mother has said her house won't sell till spring, we wouldn't have to sell the house at all; we'd be about a hundred and twenty-five thousand dollars richer. As it is, this particular repetition is bothering me more than most. I understand that each time my mother asserts that the house won't sell, she is also asserting her independence. But beliefs are powerful, and so is my mother. When I was growing up she used to tell me, "Don't tempt Fate." Now, I feel, she is instructing Fate. Making her wishes so abundantly clear to Fate that Fate will wait. And the house won't sell until my mother wills it to happen. Spring? Maybe. Or maybe never.

What I know is that we can't wait for spring. I'm worried about the winter months. I remind my mother that I'll be traveling for work. I mention the dangers in her neighborhood: a recent notice from the local police department has informed us that an alleged drug dealer is living across the street.

"I've always known something was fishy about the people in that house. And to think it is a Habitat house! Jimmy Carter should come take it away from them. Selling drugs out of one of his houses!"

I don't mention that the dealer of drugs is innocent until

proven guilty in a court of law. Her presence in the neighborhood has made my mother more willing to move.

"Why don't we visit Sunrise and see what you think?"

"Sunrise! What a name!"

I let that one go. I don't want to admit that the irony of the
name has occurred to me too. It isn't as bad as the elder housing
complex in the town where I went to high school. That one is
located at the end of Hemlock Drive.

"You could try it out for the winter. I'd feel a lot better with
you living there when I'm out of town."

"How much?" she asks again.

"Let's just see how you like it and then work out the finances, okay? Why don't we go up tomorrow?"

"I can't afford to move anywhere until I sell this place."

"Mom, I can manage the money if it seems like a good place
for you to spend the winter."

She presses me: "How much does it cost?"

"Around two thousand dollars a month."

"There's no way I can afford that on my pension."

"Once the house sells, you'll be able to afford it—and remember, it includes heat, utilities, and all your meals. In the
meantime, I can manage the money."

"Who asked you to?"

"You did."

"Bullshit! You are managing my money without my permission."

"Bullshit back to you! We opened the account together and
you signed all the paperwork."

I try to collect myself. This conversation is not going as
planned. Noreen and Suzanne had suggested that I ask my
mother to try Sunrise for the winter months. If I am able to
get my mother to make a short-term commitment, they told
me, there's a good chance I can persuade her to stay put once

she's moved in. But the timing and the unsold house complicate matters. At two thousand dollars a month, I'm lowballing the costs of Sunrise, which are closer to three thousand—several hundred dollars more than her monthly pension. It's a stretch for me to reassure my mother that she shouldn't worry about the money when I'm worrying about it most of the time.

I obsess over the costs of my mother's continued care, the sorry state of her finances, and the uncertainty of mine. My uncle Jack has offered to front the cost of assisted living until my mother's house sells. It's a generous offer, and one I wish I had the wherewithal to decline. But my mother's pension barely covers her current housing expenses, and I have no reserves of my own. When I think to the future—after my mother's house sells, after my mother is safe and ensconced in the right supported setting—I start doing the math: the proceeds from the house, combined with my mother's pension, will cover the costs of assisted living for about three years. And that assumes the costs of her care—and the level of care required—will remain relatively stable.

After those three years are up? I hope I will find a way to support her.

At the moment, it's not looking good. My writing income, if I were to divide monies received by hours spent, would come in below minimum wage. I do better with my consulting projects, but the work is not steady or consistent. There's been little of it over the past several months. I've taken advantage of the space in my schedule to complete another book, but much of my time has been focused on attending to my mother's business. I have been grateful for the flexibility, but I am now in desperate need of income. Up to my ears in debt and struggling to pay my own bills, I find it difficult to imagine how I will cover my mother's rising expenses, even three years down the road.

But I can't think about any of this now. I'm determined to

get my mother into a safe and social environment as soon as possible and to keep her secure—and with any luck, happy and healthy—for as long as possible.

"Mom, look, can we just go see the place together?"

"Oh, all right, Kathleen."

"We'll drive to Plymouth tomorrow and have dinner at Sunrise to check out the food. I'll give you a reminder call when I'm leaving my house to come get you."

"Fine, fine. I'm only doing this for you, you know."

I hold in the sigh. I hold back the words. "Thanks, Mom," I say. "I appreciate it."

Hanging up, I realize that tonight it is just Bix and me for dinner. For the first time in close to a month, I don't need to worry about making a nutritious meal that my mother will eat. And even better—I don't have to hear my mother hum while I am chopping vegetables.

I take a deep breath; it's almost like I am breathing in the silence.

I will eat leftovers tonight. I will enjoy peace, quiet, and the company of Bix. And until further notice, I will allow myself to believe that everything is going to work out fine.

Chapter Eleven

Only Child

I have more siblings than most only children do. In the six-parent blend of four first and second marriages, I am the eldest of seven children. Nine, if you count my original siblings: a brother and sister, lost before I was four years old. Combined, their time on earth was limited to a half handful of days. Maybe because there is a lot of Irish Catholic in my family, I was made aware of their brief lives by the time I was six. I'd been asking my mother for a brother or sister for a while. The source of my desire was my best friend, Bobby. I sensed the connection between Bobby and his two older sisters, and in the same way I coveted the cool toys that Bobby got on every birthday—his father worked at Hasbro—I wanted siblings just like his.

I remember sitting on the living room couch, watching my mother fold laundry, when I mentioned how helpful I would be with a new baby and how much fun we would have later, when my new brother or sister was older.

"You have a brother and a sister, Katie, but they're in Heaven." She told me their names: Paul Christopher and Seanne Marie. "You were too little to remember when I had Paul, but I bet you remember a couple of years ago, going to the hospital with me a lot to get my blood drawn?"

Yes, I remembered those trips to the hospital. My mother

and I would sit side by side in those chair-and-desk combinations like they had at the high school. She would extend her arm, palm upward, onto the desk while a nurse tied a rubber band up close to the elbow, usually mumbling about having trouble finding a good vein or mentioning how delicate my mother's arms were. I was relieved the nurse never tried to find a good vein on me. When we got home from the hospital, I remembered, my mother would wrap herself in the cobalt-blue bathrobe that showed off her eyes and put her feet up, because her ankles were so swollen.

"I was expecting your sister, Seanne, then. Your father and I didn't tell you, because we knew we had this problem with our blood types—I have something called Rh negative and he's Rh positive, and it can make it hard to have a baby together. When you were born, that was the first question I asked. 'What's her blood type?' When the doctor said 'A-positive,' I said, 'Thank God!' I was so relieved! You'll never have this problem when you have children."

I was still in kindergarten. My Rh factor seemed a distant issue to me.

"After I had Seanne, the doctor said it would be too dangerous for me to have another baby."

True, I'd asked for a sibling on more than one occasion, but the whole concept of how brothers and sisters showed up on the planet was still pretty mysterious to me. Until that moment, I had no idea that my mother's swollen ankles were in any way connected with a possible baby, and I certainly didn't get how an unknown baby girl had the potential to hurt my mom. This may have been my first experience of a conversation with my mother careening out of control. A heretofore unknown pair of siblings in heaven? My mother's life on the line because of something in her blood? Well, there was no contest between my desire for a kid sister and my need to keep my mother alive. I never raised the subject again.

My mother never dropped it. Throughout my childhood, she reminded me that my Rh positive blood type was a huge benefit, though it wasn't until we studied genetics in high school that I understood why that might be true. She mentioned my siblings routinely, and always by name, as if we had been introduced. To me, they were more like characters in a sad story ending in death—an impression reinforced by the poem that my grandmother wrote about the two tiny sibling stars in heaven. The poem—lettered in black and gold on creamy stretched silk, under glass and enclosed in a gilt-edged frame—followed us from house to house. It was around this time that my mother began collecting Hummels, boys and girls who never grew up.

In all honesty, my dead siblings, their swish-embellished poem, and especially the Hummel boys and girls have creeped me out for most of my life. But recently I find myself wishing that my angel-sibs were all grown up and living on earth instead of in heaven. It isn't that I don't feel blessed by all my late-arriving semi-siblings, but every one of them shares a mother with at least one other.

I share a mother—my mother—with none of them.

Lately, when asked how many children she has, my mother answers, "Three." I'm not sure whether she is rightly claiming three pregnancies, three labors, and three births, or whether she is blurring the dividing line between the dead and the living. I know their presence and absence has been with my mother for most of her adult life, and it seems she plans to take Paul and Seanne with her into this next phase.

I've heard plenty of stories about siblings fighting over the correct course of care for their aging parents, and more than one person has told me I am lucky to be able to make decisions without consulting with an uncooperative or unhelpful brother or sister. But even among siblings who disagree, there is typically shared care and concern for their parent's well-being.

Not only am I without full-blood siblings, I am also husbandless—never married—without children, and, for most of my taxpaying life, self-employed. Without any conscious intention, I have achieved forty-six years without traditional alliances—emotional, institutional, or financial. I don't have to wrangle with my four-year-old hyperactive son while I am untangling my mother's finances. I don't have to ask my boss for permission to take my mother to a doctor's appointment. My teenage daughter is not acting out because she is afraid of what's happening to her grandmother, and my relationship with my husband is not strained by the weight of my mother's illness. On the other hand, I am entirely dependent on my own wits to keep myself fed and sheltered, and I am without the distraction, relief, buffer, and support of family life. When my mother is gone—lost to death or the final phase of her forgetting—I will be the sole survivor of my family of origin, and without a family of my origination. Only—and alone.

෴

Though always present, onlyness is not a state I cultivate. From my first friend, Bobby, I learned it is possible to fight and make up. I can't remember how many times we were told to "just shake hands" discovering that once we did, we were, indeed, friends again. From Bobby I learned, too, that it was possible to be friends long-distance—even in an era that required letter writing to stay in touch. My first friendship taught me one more thing: that it is possible for a girl to be friends with a boy without being boyfriend and girlfriend. I've since read that early friendships between girls and boys change the way we interact as men and women, and despite my single state, I believe the changes are ultimately for the better. And the last time I heard from his older sister, Bobby was happily married with children. So I cannot blame my singleness on my first true friend.

When my parents split up, my mother and I moved from our house in Rhode Island to a damp basement apartment in Massachusetts. A year later, we moved again, into a small house a couple of towns away. We stayed there for three years, until my mother married Richard, when we moved one more time. Here are the childhood mathematics: three elementary schools in three different towns; two years of junior high; another move, another town; high school. For me, an ability to make friends was a requisite survival tool.

In high school, I met Cindy. Our friendship formed in our freshman year as we walked together from geometry class to the band room for the last period of the day. She played clarinet, but she wasn't a music geek. An athlete, she played a mean defense on the field hockey team. Cindy had beautiful, long red-blonde hair, and she was part of a clique whose members, while not exactly "cool," were confident, outgoing, connected, and accepted. I remember a few years ago mentioning to Cindy's daughter that her mother was one of the popular kids in high school, and Brooke was incredulous. Her entirely uncool mom was popular in high school? I had to clarify: popular in the wholesome set—she played in the band, after all—but Cindy's reach was far and broad. It still is. Cindy talked me into going to the only class reunion I have attended—our tenth. This coming year will be our thirtieth, and I plan to stay home. But I will look forward to hearing all about it from my longtime, true, and forever friend, Cindy.

From high school into college, from college into my early

working life, connections were made and friends were found. Over the passage of years, some friendships lost momentum, but more were sealed by time. I am surrounded, if not by immediate, blood relations, by a network of strong ties and close relationships. My friends are my executive board, my cheerleaders, my tribe. In rough chronological order of meeting: Cindy, Mimi, Harry, Bruce, Tony, Tom, Lara, Katrina, Shannon, Anne.

And Tina. We've known each other just eight years, but Tina and I have a depth of understanding and connection that defies any space or time. "Through a mutual friend," we answer when we are asked, "How did you meet?" The uncut story of our meeting is more complicated. I'd heard about Tina for years before I met her—from my longtime colleague Eric, who was also Tina's adoring boyfriend. She worked for American Airlines; Eric worked for the airport division of one of my regular clients at the time, Waterstone's Booksellers. He and I were working to prepare five bookstores in time for the opening of a giant new airport in Hong Kong when Eric—just thirty-three—suffered a major heart attack. I first laid eyes on Tina at the old Hong Kong airport. She was big-eyed and beautiful, looking flight-attendant fresh after spending twenty hours in the air and crossing continents to reach her sweetheart's bedside. Eric had lost consciousness in the time it took to locate Tina and get her to Hong Kong, but I hoped he sensed her presence, hoped that some part of Eric knew that his mother and his brother had traveled from Boston to be with him, that I was still there too. Eric would pass away—too young and too far away from home—but he would not die alone.

Tina, who was based in Boston, came to visit me several times that summer. We talked late into the night as she tried to unravel what had happened. She was eager for the details I could supply, and I was eager to be with someone who had shared the experience in Hong Kong. Perhaps because our friendship was born under such difficult circumstances, it seems to me to have a sense of destiny to it—or rightness. I cannot imagine my life now without Tina in it. We are the witnesses for the largeness of each other's lives. We comfort each other; we laugh together. We bodysurf in summertime, sip green tea and eat dark chocolate in wintertime, and talk on the phone pretty much every day she isn't flying.

Three years after Eric died, Tina began talking about another flight attendant; he was funny, smart, and had—her words, now—*prominent eyebrows*. A year ago, Tina married Jonathan in a small ceremony at City Hall. That morning we visited a hair salon, where the stylist worked Tina's thick, curly locks into a too-tall French twist. Back at her house, an hour before the ceremony, Tina had a bridal meltdown. "I look like a Conehead!" She began to pull at her hair. "You have to fix this!" It was a command that I did my best to obey. In the wedding photos, Tina's hair—swept up and strewn with tiny white flowers salvaged from her bouquet to cover up my inexpert use of bobby pins—looks almost as lovely as she does.

If friends are chosen family, Tina and Cindy may save me from my only-child status. Their personalities, their ways of being in the world—they couldn't be more different. But Cindy, like Tina, has experienced a profound and premature loss—in Cindy's case, her husband at the age of forty to pancreatic cancer. For Cindy, as for Tina, I was nearby, helping and yet helpless in the face of what seemed like a series of horrific mistakes on the part of the universe.

I wonder if heartbreak is the prerequisite for empathy. Do we have to feel our own hearts break open before we can be present for the heartbreak of another? Cindy, Tina—they both have the capacity to show up for me now. Is it just who they are, or is it where they have been, what they have experienced, what they have lost, and how they have lived beyond their losses?

Tina visits from New Hampshire, where she and Jonathan have a house now. She comes to lunch with me and my mother. She smiles and engages with her, and as Tina listens to my mother repeat herself, she remains charming, interested all over again. "What a lovely girl," my mother says to me when Tina excuses herself to use the restroom.

Cindy, who lives in New Jersey, checks in by phone, always willing to listen as I share the latest about my mother. "I feel so bad for you," she says. In my more noble moments, I don't want to be the object of Cindy's sympathy. I want her to save it up for my mother. But I don't have to summon up nobility for the sake of my oldest friend.

I am safe with Cindy. And with Tina too, who understands that I feel conflicted and guilty about moving forward with my mom. "Getting your mother into assisted living is the best thing you can do for her," she assures me—and reassures me every time she senses I need to hear it again. In the midst of my looking out for my mother, my dearest sister-friends will be looking out for me.

✍

Then why do I feel so alone? Is it that word again—*Alzheimer's*? Or the combination of words: *My mother has Alzheimer's*. I have heard the silence that follows the declaration, the extra two-beat pause that signals discomfort. Health care professionals respond with a solemn nod. Friends, acquaintances, even strangers weigh in with ideas and information, all designed to help save me from the same fate. Jack and Rosemary, my mother's siblings and my closest advisers on my mother's care, never speak the word aloud. Rosemary refers to my mother's "issues," and Jack focuses on her "requirements for care." I know their resistance may be rooted in their experience with Nana. It can't be easy to be reminded of the last few years of your mother's life when you are speaking of your own sister.

The reluctance of Rose, Jack, and others to name this disease—the same reluctance I felt just weeks ago—makes me that much more determined to brand it: *Alzheimer's.* Some sort of self-inflicted aversion therapy, perhaps—and at the same time, a perverse test for others in my life. I need people now who can handle the reality of this situation. I have no time for ambiguity and little room for those who, in fearing for themselves, cannot find empathy for my mother. I am impatient. And I am fierce, protective, like a mother lion. I know that I am about to set in motion a series of events that will not make my mother happy. But I need the support of someone—or better, several someones—who understand I am doing the best I can and that doing this particular best is not easy. I need these someones to understand, too, that I have to talk about what's happening. The weather no longer interests me.

Yes, I want to say, it is scary for all of us. But imagine how scary it is to be my mother. As I wash the dishes for the fourth time today, I think about all the tasks I do on autopilot. And I wonder: when did my mother forget how to do the dishes? She has a dishwasher. Was there a time—back when she could remember where to put the soap and how to load the machine, a time before she lost her sequencing ability—when she washed and rewashed the dishes, unable to remember or ascertain whether they were dirty or clean? And would she still remember how to do the dishes if, like me, she had been doing them by hand day after day, year after year?

It's a crazy thing to contemplate, but the mundane tasks are what trip my mother up. She's able to fake the conversation, and her vocabulary—unlike many patients with dementia—has barely suffered. It's all those years of teaching English. But housecleaning? Never her strong suit, and perhaps, for her, not worth the effort now to fake. Since I stepped across her threshold over a year ago, I have come to understand that the mess inside was not a product of not caring or depression, but rather of forgetting. I realize there is a good chance my mother cannot remember how to keep things tidy. The coffee grounds all over the counter are a symptom of her disease and an indication that something she has done every day of her adult life—making her morning coffee—is a task that now eludes her. "It doesn't work right anymore," she says about the machine, but what she is really saying is, "I don't work right anymore. And I'm scared."

I finish the dishes and call Suzanne. As much comfort and support as they can give me, Cindy and Tina have families, lives, and mothers of their own—and they aren't exactly down the street. My uncle Jack is willing to offer financial and logistical support, and my aunt Rosemary wants the best for my mom and offers moral support to me, but they too are at a distance. I need someone on the ground, nearby, and someone who has no trouble saying the A-word out loud.

"My mother agreed to move to Sunrise for the winter, and her move-in date is less than a week away," I tell Suzanne. "I've been to her house three times with the intention of helping her figure out what to take, but we get nowhere. I know I need to push her, but she gets so hostile. And I'm not sure her hating me is going to make this easier. On the other hand, making her happy means not moving her into Sunrise—and . . ."

"And she does need to move; it's the best scenario for her, and for you, too. How can I help?"

"Can I hire you—even just to help us through this transition?"

"Of course. It will be a lot easier for me to do than it is for you."

"You mean she's less likely to accuse you of putting her away, or tell you this isn't the way a good daughter treats her mother?"

Suzanne chuckles. "Yes, I'll keep it very professional. I'll explain I'm there to help her get ready for the move. I'll bring little Post-its and we'll label the things she wants to take—mostly pictures and maybe a chair or two. You're borrowing a bed from Sunrise, so we don't need to worry about that. Who will be helping you move?"

"My uncle—my mother's brother, Jack. We're renting a van. Tuesday."

"I can't be there on Tuesday, but I'll be up at Sunrise on Wednesday to do some staff training, and I'll be sure to check on your mother then. We can speak Wednesday night or Thursday if you like."

"That would be great."

"Don't worry, Kate," she says. "I'll go over on Monday, and we'll get this done."

But I am worried. About my mother; about the extra money I've decided to spend on Suzanne. About how long my mother's house might sit empty and on the market. About borrowing—and paying back—the money for the assisted living expenses from Jack. About getting enough work to pay my own bills. About maintaining my calm and sureness with my mother, even as I question every move I am making on her behalf. About how I will ever get us through this. About a million and a half other things. My small world weighs heavy on my shoulders.

"Kate?" Suzanne says. "You're not alone." Not for the first

time or the last time, she has read my mind. When she came to the house, Suzanne told me I never had to be alone in this, and I wasn't sure what she meant. I still wonder whether she is trying to give me a more cosmic message, but I know that she is also telling me I can choose—and have chosen—to ask for help and support from my friends, from my mother's family, and even from professionals like her.

Only—yes, and sometimes lonely. But not alone.

Chapter Twelve

Life Inside

Have I sent my mother to an elder prison packed with card-playing, antisocial inmates? That's what she would have me believe. I'm inclined to think it isn't as bad as that. Even so, I am not at all certain that I have done the right thing. I fret and worry about her capacity to settle in. She snarls at me and does her best to make me feel like a horrible person. We're twenty-seven hours into my mother's stay at Sunrise, and it seems neither one of us is adapting too well.

Moments ago, my mother hung up on me after making this subtle distinction: "Just so you know—I don't hate you for sending me here. But I do dislike you intensely."

Our phone call hadn't begun well, either.

"What you and my brother have done to me is unspeakable—packing me up and carting me off to this place. And where is my car? I need my car! This place is a prison. *A prison.* You sent me to a prison."

"Mom, you've only been there a day—"

"A day? I've been here for weeks! And I hate it every day."

For a minute I think my mother is being overdramatic to prove her point, but then I remember that lately my mother's sense of time has gone askew. Distance too. "Are we there yet?" she'll ask me, fifteen minutes into the journey to a family gathering at Jack's. It's a drive we've made for years, and it takes two hours without cigarette breaks. "Why does my brother live so damn far away?"

My mother has been at Sunrise for a night and a day, but it feels to her as if she has been there for several weeks. At this rate of time conversion, we could be in for a very long winter of assisted living.

Three days ago—the day before the big move—Suzanne knocked on my mother's front door, clipboard and pad of sticky notes in hand. "I wouldn't say that your mother is happy about going to Sunrise, but she understands it's happening," she reported back to me that evening. "I reminded her that you'd be away on projects a lot this winter. While we were deciding what she would take with her, I reinforced that she would be much happier at Sunrise than she would be staying alone in her neighborhood."

"And she was okay—I mean she was willing to participate in making the decisions with you?"

"I printed out the list you e-mailed me and used that as a guide. She passed on some things you suggested, and she decided to take some things you hadn't mentioned. We labeled everything she wants to take with Post-it notes. Overall, I'd say your mother was cooperative."

On moving day, *cooperative* was not the operative word. Whether my mother had forgotten she had agreed to go to Sunrise or had just decided to play it that way, she did her level best to make it difficult for the moving team: my uncle Jack, my friend Shannon, and me. Shannon is a landscape designer with a pickup truck and a light schedule in the wintertime. As it turned out, we didn't need Shannon's truck, but her strong back and upbeat attitude were much appreciated. Shannon and my mother have met on several occasions, but she isn't family. I was hoping that her third-party presence might help dispel my mother's inevitable anger toward me and Jack—or at least keep it at bay. I knew that having a good friend in tow would make me feel better too. And I thought that three would be better than two when it came to some of the heavier items. Jack tends to think he's about half his age, and I didn't want to be responsible for too many strained muscles.

Jack, Shannon, and I were an excellent moving team, as it turned out. We moved clothing, furniture, lamps, and boxes of knickknacks through the front door and into the rented van. We worked quickly and with a minimum of mishaps. Meanwhile my mother sat, immoveable, on the loveseat in her living room, steaming as much as smoking. "You have no right to come into my house and just take things out of it!" she hissed at Jack. He ignored her.

"Mom, I noticed you didn't tag this print, but I know you love it. Don't you want to take it with you?" I was trying redirection, a technique Suzanne had suggested would come in handy.

"I never agreed to go anywhere. You have some nerve to just put me wherever you want me. Wherever it's convenient for you!"

"Mom, remember—we visited Sunrise together, and you liked it the best of the places we looked at. I am not *putting* you anywhere."

She stamped out her cigarette and lit another.

"So the picture, Mom. Would you like to take it?"

"I don't give a goddamn. You're deciding everything else for me. You might as well decide that too. You and Jack. Who the hell does he think he is?"

"Let's take this. I think it will look nice in your new place."

Jack and Shannon rode in the van; my mother rode with me. We were maybe seven minutes from her driveway when my mother said, "I had no idea this place was so far away."

I reassured her that Sunrise wasn't far away, thirty-five or forty minutes from my front door, that I'd be able to visit often when I wasn't out of town. Suzanne has suggested that I continue to remind my mother I will be working off-Cape a lot in the coming months. My mother, when she thinks of me away on business, is more willing to move out of her drug-dealing neighborhood. In fact, I have too little work lined up this winter. For better or worse, my recent focus has been on my mother's business rather than my own. But if I'm going to feel comfortable about taking on projects that demand travel, I need to know my mother is safe and cared for.

"We've been in the car at least an hour. My fanny is killing me."

"That's because you don't have enough padding on your skinny butt." This is a regular topic of conversation. My mother is proud of her skinny body and her tiny butt, despite the painful inconvenience of sitting on it. "Now if you had my butt . . ."

She laughed. It was a predictable routine—a comic bit that we do together. She doesn't want my butt any more than I want hers. She says I have a "Sliney body," which means I am proportioned more like my grandmother, while my mom has a "Ford body," slender like her father's. According to my mother, the only thing that saves me is that I got the "Whouley height," thus stretching my bulk across a taller frame. My too-skinny mother's assessments of my too-big body parts can get on my nerves, but at that moment I was happy to steer the conversation away from the matter, and the destination, at hand.

At last we pulled into the driveway of Sunrise, Jack and Shannon right behind us. "*Sunrise*," my mother read aloud. "What a name. Who do they think they're kidding?"

Evidently, a little more than a day later, not my mother.

"Mom, I know it feels like you've been there longer, but it's only been a day. Let's give the place a chance. Just for the winter, so you're safe while I'm traveling. And maybe tomorrow will be better. When you get to know more people—"

"What people? Everyone keeps to themselves here. They just come out of their rooms to eat. That's it."

"There's a bulletin board right outside your room where they post the daily activities. Maybe you can see what's happening tomorrow."

"Activities! Bridge, bridge, bridge and bridge, and I don't play bridge." We'd moved into familiar territory. For months my mother has claimed that she checked out the activities at the senior center in her town and discovered that all they did there was play bridge.

"Mom, when I checked the calendar yesterday, I didn't even see bridge listed. Just have a look, okay?"

Her voice softened. "It's lonely here."

"I was thinking I could come visit Friday. We could hang some pictures, get your place set up."

"Oh, that would be nice." She sounded like she meant it.

"Today's Wednesday, so that will be two days from now." Even before my mother's trouble with time and distance, she has needed help with the days of the week. Since she retired, she has been loathe to consult a calendar. She thinks calendars are universally ugly and unworthy of wall space.

"Two days," she repeated. "Will you bring my car?"

"Mom, your car's in the shop, remember? There is something wrong with it. It can't be driven."

"I can't stay here without a car! You might as well put me in prison. You have put me in prison! This place is *a prison*!"

✑

Suzanne's well-timed e-mail arrives moments after my mother's declaration of intense dislike.

Just a brief note to let you know I looked in on your mom a few times yesterday. She most definitely remembered me, and though there was a bit of sarcasm in her voice about not wanting to be at Sunrise, each time I saw her, she was well engaged in socializing with Marilyn and some of the other ladies. When she mentioned to them that she didn't like the fact that her family just put her things in a truck and brought her to Sunrise, they all laughed and one of them said, "How else do you think they would have gotten you to come? You'll get over it, dear. This will become like home to you very soon." Being able to discuss how she feels with her peers and getting such positive feedback from them will help ease her transition. The constant availability of coffee right outside her door doesn't hurt either. Now if we can just curb the cigarette smoking, all else will fall into place.

I'm relieved to hear that contrary to my mother's own assessment of the situation, she is socializing and making friends. But the combination of guilt and regret and sadness and just sheer worry for my mother's well-being renders me sleepless again tonight. In what might be a perverse act of self-preservation, my worries crystallize into one single concern: what if my mother goes out for an evening cigarette and gets locked out?

I picture her with that big blue parka that she never zips up, going out for her last smoke of the night and forgetting that they lock the door at seven, forgetting that she can ring the buzzer to get back in.

Is this how you keep your mother safe? the voice of guilt asks me, sometime in the wee hours. My exhaustion feeds the fear, strengthens the power of that voice. I find myself walking through any number of horrific scenarios. After seven, there would be no one at the reception desk to notice my mother's departure. And Sunrise, so far as I know, isn't the sort of place that does bed checks. And what would my mother do if she were locked out? Decide, in a fit of pique, to leave the damn place, take a walk down the long driveway, parka unzipped, gloveless, and wearing her slippers? When would they discover her missing? At breakfast? Even later?

In the morning, I call to check on my mother's whereabouts. "She's right here in the lobby, having some coffee with the girls. Would you like to speak to her?" Sandy, the mainstay at the front desk, knows there's been a delay in getting my mother's room phone working.

"I would, but before I do, can I ask you something?" I explain to the always-kind receptionist that I am worried about my mother, her smoking, the buzzer, the locked doors.

"Why don't you call back tonight, just before seven, and talk to the night staff? Your mom isn't the only smoker, so I bet they have it worked out. Do you want me to leave a note?"

"Thanks—I'll call back later—but let me say a quick hello to my mom, if you don't mind."

"Hello, Kathleen," my mother says when she comes to the phone. If she's using my full name, my mother is either annoyed with me or feeling mischievous and wanting me to think she is annoyed. I'm guessing it is the former, but still, I plow ahead as if everything is fine.

"Hi, Mom. How was breakfast?"

"Too early," she says. "They make such a racket getting it ready. I'm awake whether I want to be or not."

"Well, how's the coffee?" I ask her.

"You know, the coffee is good."

In the days and nights that follow, I will hold on to the fact that my mother likes the coffee at Sunrise. I will begin to sleep at night, comforted by the knowledge that the night supervisor has equipped my mother's door frame with a hook-and-paper-clip creation that signifies whether my mother is in or out. I will be assured that everyone on the night staff makes a point of checking the paper clip—and my mother's room. And in the not too distant future, I will learn that my mother has her last cigarette at ten of seven, just before the doors are locked for the night. She has come to believe that is just one more injustice in the Sunrise prison system, and I let her live with that belief. Again and again, I am equally surprised by what my mother re-members—is able to retain and organize—and by what she for-gets or doesn't understand. She forgets she can use the buzzer after seven, but she remembers, always, to get out for that last cigarette of the night just before the doors are locked.

My mother will continue to complain about being in prison. She will continue to ask for her car. She will continue to be angry with me for "sending" her to Sunrise. I will visit at least once a week, and we will develop a ritual of supply runs to CVS, where my mother stocks up on snacks, buys the occasional greeting card, surveys the lipsticks and nail polishes, and always buys a carton of Benson & Hedges Lights. We will eat out, mostly at the Ninety Nine Restaurant, where, after scanning the menu, my mother will ask me, "What do I like?"

"The teriyaki chicken is one of your favorites. Or when you're in the mood for seafood, you like the fish and chips."

When the waitress comes, my mother will smile at her before she looks at me and asks, "What did I decide to get, Katie?"

"You were thinking of ordering the teriyaki chicken."

"Right. I like that. I'll have teriyaki chicken."

"That comes with rice and your choice of vegetable."

"No rice. I'd like french fries, please."

"Fries instead of rice. No problem," says the waitress. "Now for your vegetable . . ." She reels off a list.

"I'd like french fries."

"Double fries," I clarify for my mother and the waitress. It should be noted here that when my mother orders fish and chips, she also goes for double fries, no coleslaw.

"Yes. What I don't eat, I'll take with me," she tells the waitress. We will put the leftovers in the minifridge that my uncle Jack has provided for my mom's room. The following week, I will dump out the white Styrofoam container of fries and replace it with another. My mother rarely opens her fridge and has little awareness of its contents. But it is important to her; having a fridge in her room gives her status among her fellow residents, who sometimes ask to put something in it—and so I am not surprised when I open the fridge one week to find a bouquet of fruit that was sent to my mother's new friend, Josie. Josie's memory is worse than my mother's, and the fruit, although cold, is untouched and looking a little past peak.

My visits are predictable and, I hope, reassuring to my mother. We have moments when I feel like all is well, or as well as it can be between us. But as soon as we turn back into the driveway of Sunrise, my mother's mood shifts; she becomes angry at me all over again.

"Oh, here we are back at prison!"

"Oh, Mom. It's not that bad—"

"You have no idea! You don't know what it's like to live with a bunch of strangers."

"But Mom, you have friends here now. Josie, Marilyn . . ." I start naming names.

"Josie's a nice lady, but Marilyn—she's mean."

"Mean?" The first time my mother declares that Marilyn is mean, I don't believe her. That nice lady who was looking forward to being my mother's buddy? Mean? In time I will discover that Marilyn is not always the kind, sweet lady that she was the day I visited Sunrise. But my mother's biggest problem with Marilyn, I will learn, is that she likes to play cards, and, according to my mother, she yells at anyone who makes a mistake.

The problem is eventually resolved: "Marilyn threw me out of the poker game and told me she would never play cards with me again."

"Well, from what I understand, Marilyn is sometimes in a lot of pain. When she isn't feeling well, she behaves badly. But you have Josie and the older lady from upstairs, Maria— and Geri, right on your floor, seems nice. You've met and made friends with a lot more people than you would have if you were spending the winter on the Cape."

"But I'd rather be there! You had no right to send me here!"

"I didn't send you here. Remember? We looked at a few places together, and you chose Sunrise—"

"I *chose* this place? Well I must have been *crazy*. Nuts! *Cuckoo!*"

"I'm going let you out at the door, and then I'll go park. Maybe you want to have a cigarette," I suggest.

Her tone lightens. "I would love to have a cigarette."

I have a millisecond of hopefulness that our visit will end on an up-note before my mother shifts her tone. "Yes, I would love to have a cigarette before the wardens lock us up for the night."

Chapter Thirteen

Romper Room

I was born and baptized into the Catholic Church, but I operate in the world as a disciple of *Romper Room*. To this day, I believe that *please* and *thank you* really are the magic words; I do my best to live life as a Do-Bee (rather than a Don't-Bee) and to follow the Golden Rule. I can even trace my faith in the inexplicable to the *Romper Room* closing ritual. Toward the end of each show, the hostess, Miss Jeanne, would pick up something that looked like a magnifier without the glass—circular and the size of an extra-large hand mirror. "I see Jimmy, and I see Laura," she would begin, each day reciting a different list of the kids she saw out there, on the other side of the TV. I hoped one day she would see me, but I was undisturbed, though a bit disappointed, when she didn't call my name.

One might argue that it was my early exposure to Catholicism that made me open to the mystic elements of *Romper Room*. I wouldn't preclude that possibility. As a disciple of *Romper Room*, I am not in the business of precluding any possibilities. I am a practicing adherent of the Doctrine of the Possible. It's a helpful theology for the writer in me, though it sometimes trips up the woman. More than once in my life, I have seen the possibility in a project or the potential of a person, only to discover that the present reality is inalterable. What I see, in these cases, is not what I get.

Still, I am content living life with the hope that we can move beyond ourselves, believing our world is mutable, that we can make changes large and small, that one day fewer people will be hungry or angry or caught in the crossfire of war. At the same time—and this might be writer's theology too—I am fascinated by the human predicament, by our flaws, our limitations—by the fact that we are here at all.

I don't recall much talk of souls on *Romper Room*, but I do believe we have them—or more accurately, they have us. This particular tenet in my personal theology may be attributed as easily to my Catholic roots as to my collegiate encounters with Aristotle, or to the fact that I read *The Seat of the Soul* even before Oprah discovered Gary Zukav. I believe—or at the least, I believe it is possible—that our souls transcend our human bodies, that we possess an essence that comes and goes and comes again, matching up with a new body, a new personality, a new time.

In my worldview, it is possible that our souls elect how and when to become incarnate, though I have trouble embracing the notion that souls elect lifetimes of enduring hardship, starvation, abject poverty, or abuse. I don't think it is as simple as "That's their karma," which sounds to me like an excuse not to worry about the rest of the world. I do believe there is some element of karma at work in our lives, but I also believe—strongly—that we are blessed with free will, that the choices we make influence any destiny we might have attached to us. Our intentions matter, as do our actions; though I am disinclined to presume that I can single-mindedly make things go my way—not only because there are so many of us on the planet with ever-competing desires, but because I believe there is a force larger than all of us. I'm not too worried about who or what that force might be. I'm just relieved to know that He, She, or It is not I.

Still, I do have some modicum of control in my own domain, most notably in the way I interact with myself and others. In this personal arena, the Golden Rule holds up for me as an awfully good basis for right behavior—at least human to human. It suggests that karmic awareness is trumped by compassion. There's no guarantee that our good actions will consistently and only beget good, nor is there any certainty that the bad guys get theirs in the end. By doing unto others as we would have others do unto us, we're simply doing the right thing.

While I was in Hong Kong eight years ago, I sent a few group e-mails asking for prayers and good intentions on my colleague Eric's behalf. I told his story, and in that way I told mine. I asked friends for their support as I did my best to support Eric and, later, Tina and Eric's family. "Gee, I didn't know you were that close," more than one person observed. In their minds, I was acting the way one would act on behalf of a family member, or maybe a best friend. In my mind, I did for Eric only what I would hope someone might do for me, only what seemed appropriate for one compassionate being to do for another.

Likewise with my mother. "You and your mother are so close," people have said to me, presumably basing this observation on the fact that I have not abandoned her to danger and confusion, that I have cared for and protected her from harm. In fact, our relationship—complex and not always easy—has never been what I would call close. For a good portion of my childhood, my mother was barely there—distracted by disappointment and the demands of a volatile second husband, finding solace and her identity in her work outside the home. For most of my twenties and good chunk of my thirties, I found myself at odds with my mother. She was often critical, sarcastic, and sometimes just plain mean. I felt as though I needed to shield myself, sharing less and less of my life with her. She met my retreat with repeated advances. She was capable of kind words, but more often she called on her verbal prowess to fashion creative, biting remarks.

We were stuck in a seemingly endless cycle of hurt and anger, dotted with occasional moments of connection that gave me hope. It took me years to see that the trouble in our relationship could be traced to my mother's increasing use, and eventual overuse, of alcohol. When I finally figured it out, I felt angry and betrayed. *How could she? After all we've been through?* Time and a support group helped me to understand that my mom could not control her drinking, nor could I. Still, I organized an intervention—which failed miserably. A few years later she was hospitalized and from there sent to an inpatient rehab. That's when my mother came to live with me. Her verbal cruelty abated considerably when she stopped drinking, and we began to forge a new relationship. We discovered we could enjoy each other's company. We had a run of nearly ten good years before the dementia showed up. The anger that now accompanies my mother's illness feels uncomfortably familiar— and deeply disheartening.

I am not caring for my mother because we are in close, enviable harmony. No. In choosing now to care for my mother, I am choosing to do what I would hope some kindhearted person might one day do for me. It is less about the fact that my mother is my mother—in truth, forgetting our long history makes it easier for me to relate to her—and more about the fact that my mother is a fellow human being in need of my help.

The irony is that by attending to my mother in this time of her need, I've learned to see her. To see her outside of the tangled relationship between us; to see her in her vulnerability and her fear, and to enjoy her unfailing sense of humor. At Sunrise she is already beloved. Her fellow residents come to sit at her table in the lobby; they laugh at her sardonic wit. They accept her, welcome her, and not infrequently stop me in the hall to tell me what a wonderful person she is. My mother—despite the picture she paints for me—is, more often than not, socializing. Even when she sits outside to have a cigarette, she ends up in conversation—with staff and, on more than one occasion, with someone on the way to a job interview. She is a source for not only humor but also information—until she forgets it, or forgets that she has already told the story. Which is fine in this setting, because most of her comrades have forgotten that they've heard it before.

In seeing my mother as a person—released from her long-standing role—I have come to appreciate her so much more. I see her sadness, her grief. I understand, on some level unconnected to me, that the loss of two children was devastating to her. I see that the abuses of her second marriage have scarred her as they have me. And I see that the failure of her first marriage—to my father, whom she loved—broke her heart. When I am particularly good at seeing her, I imagine her as a child, asthmatic before there were effective medications: sick and gasping for breath on the bad days, and walking with her father to the corner drugstore on the good days, where he would treat her to a hot fudge sundae. The loss of her father when she was sixteen, I understand now, was the first in a series of unspeakable losses in my mother's life. She has not had an easy time.

When I contemplate my mother's past and present, my thoughts wander to the composition and desires of her soul. Was her life journey initiated by her eternal soul? Or were there times when her this-life personality overruled the impulses of her soul? And how and where do I fit in? Some spiritual thinkers say that souls can travel in groups, or "soul families," and that we will find each other in our lifetimes and on some level be able to recognize each other. While I have felt that glimmer of recognition with others on the planet, I have never felt that connection with my mother. My mother's soul has always been a stranger to mine. This is not, in itself, a bad thing, but I've sometimes wished for a stronger, deeper connection to my right-now mom.

My wish: granted. I have come to care for my mother's body and mind—and in this way have forged a connection soul to soul. And I see that even on the level of personality, we have more in common than I may have imagined. "Keep on keepin' on" was one of my mother's expressions. And in the face of loss and disappointment, that is exactly what she did. She forged ahead. Often as a woman alone. She didn't tell me to do the same, but she showed me how.

It's still complicated, and there are times when I want to curse right back at her when she calls me on the phone just to swear at me. And I absolutely question the wisdom of whatever higher power it is that allows human brains to lose their capacity in such insidious ways. Years and years ago, I read that what we think of as dementia is actually the symptom of soul-wandering. The soul, preparing to depart, begins leaving the body for short intervals, and these absences lead to the confusion of the mind and lack of orientation in the body that typify Alzheimer's. Medicine and neuroscience explain Alzheimer's in more concrete terms: brain plaque, lesions, missing synapses, neurotransmitters unable to connect over the deteriorating surface of the brain.

The science makes plenty of sense to me when it comes to the physical roots of dementia, but I also like the idea of our souls taking mini vacations. At the same time, I've grown uncomfortable when I hear folks say, referring to someone with

Alzheimer's or another form of dementia, "She just isn't herself anymore," or worse, "He's just not there." I know my mother has not yet reached the most debilitating phase of this disease, and certainly I am no expert in all this. But my mother, the fellow human being—the other I can do unto—she is still there.

Unless her physical ailments take her first, my mother will pass through this middle stage and into the late stage of Alzheimer's disease. She will cease to recognize me as her daughter. I've heard other caregivers talk about how difficult this is, how sad, but I just don't see it that way. It doesn't really matter who I am to her, and it barely matters who she is to me. What matters is that she *is;* that she is safe and maybe even happy wherever she and her soul go gallivanting.

I can recall that my grandmother, late in her life, would become confused about my identity. I was in my early twenties, and I fought hard to help her place me correctly as her granddaughter. I recorded my voice, and the voices of all her children and grandchildren, and gave her a little tape recorder so she could listen and remember. I recorded myself playing the flute too, and whenever she heard the music, she would light up. "That's Katie!" she would say. And a moment later, "That's you!" She'd smile, proud of her ability to make the connection, before she would go back to the music, listening intently.

If and when my mother reaches the point that she thinks I am her sister or her mother, or even just a kindhearted visitor, I may bring her music too. But I'll do it not to prompt recognition, but just because I know she would enjoy listening. These many years later, I see that I was the only one disturbed when Nana didn't recognize me. My grandmother was content having a lovely chat with that nice young woman who came to visit her.

Alzheimer's has been called "the long goodbye," because you lose the person little by little over a period of years. Only months ago, I thought that was awful, tragic. But now I am beginning to believe there is new possibility even in the midst of loss. In forgetting, we are offered an opportunity to forgive. Everything that's old is new again. And everything that's new— on the good days—reminds us only of this: we are human, we are dear to each other, and we are here, now. And even for a *Romper Room* adherent of the Doctrine of the Possible, that is— possibly—enough.

Chapter Fourteen

Wintering

Serendipity arrives with an Irish accent.

"Sure you'll have a cuppa." Fionah nods in the direction of her traveling teakettle and hands me a mug. I sit down at my mother's kitchen table as my hostess cuts a no-fuss cheese omelet in half and presents me with a plate. Generally I'm not a big egg-eater, but on the other hand, I'm unaccustomed to any breakfast served in my mother's kitchen. Mom was always a coffee-and-cigarettes kind of morning person. Before I turned three, I mastered raisin toast slathered with oleo and sprinkled with cinnamon sugar—the favored breakfast of my childhood.

Fionah, on the other hand, believes in protein to begin the day. And I have to admit I am already growing spoiled by her belief system. It's been just thirteen days since we met—introduced at a dinner arranged by my friend Anne—and eight days since she's moved into my mother's place. My invitation was impulsive. I learned over dinner that Fionah was looking for a winter hideaway to work on her music. I knew my mother's place would soon be empty. I told Fionah it was hers, so long as she was comfortable with the uncertainty of living in a house that was on the market.

"Rent-free, of course," I clarified.

"Oh my, but can you be serious, Kate? Sure I'd pay you—"

"No, you wouldn't. I'll need about a week or so to do some clearing and cleaning—and maybe some painting—before you move in."

"Do you think I'm going to let you do all that work just so I can move in and not pay you the rent? Sure I'll help you."

"No—you don't understand. My mother is a heavy smoker, and the house reeks. It needs a good cleaning and airing out. You wouldn't want to move in right away."

Fionah made a dismissive *chhssh* sound that I would come to recognize. "I'm the youngest of seven children, and I went to Catholic boarding school. I can sleep anywhere."

In eight days' time, I've learned that Fionah is indomitable—energetic, uncomplaining, and eager for a project. The first week, we threw stuff out. Not just old papers and mildewed books, but also small pieces of cheap furniture, throw pillows, rugs—anything that was either so covered in tar or so discolored by nicotine that we deemed it unsalvageable. Everything else we scrubbed, ran through the dishwasher, or threw into the washing machine. At first I felt invigorated by the clearing and cleaning. But by day five I was deflated. I felt confronted by an inescapable fact: this is what you do after people *die*. Deciding what to keep and what to toss, going through papers. Surrounded by the detritus of my mother's life—while she was still living it elsewhere. It felt all wrong.

"Please God," Fionah began, and for a moment I thought she was praying. "It's better to do this work now, Kate. You'll be relieved of it later. The same with the house. You'll be happy to be free of it."

∽

We fill the dumpster that fills the driveway, and we work to clear the surfaces. This means hand-washing and packing up my mother's Hummels—in an odd twist, she took none of her creepy porcelain children to Sunrise—and organizing the cabinets to accommodate the overload of assorted knickknacks. The hundred-odd Santas in my mother's unofficial collection didn't come downstairs for the holidays this year; they are in the attic with all the Christmas decorations. I know we'll have to deal with them eventually, but for now we let them be. The ultimate goal of this clearing operation is to make the house more saleable. The attic can wait.

We work outward from the center of every room, eventually reaching the closets. The one in my mother's bedroom, with its sagging center pole, is easy. She never used it. But the closet in my mother's den is a larger challenge. The doors have been removed to accommodate a large pine armoire housing my mother's winter sweaters, an assortment of lace curtains, and some old dishes and vases that were once my grandmother's. Careful excavation on either side of the armoire reveals a wooden Halloween witch the size of a toddler, painted in blacks and oranges and topped with an inexplicable straw hat; a fistful of curtain rods; two giant ceramic bunnies with flowers on their tummies; a portable vacuum cleaner; a toilet plunger; and a couple of rag rugs.

There is a soft-sided leatherette suitcase under the rugs. It's the largest piece from the set my mother bought for me on her Sunoco card when I went off to college. Dragging it into the room and unzipping it, I sift through the contents: old tax returns, retirement cards, letters, cancelled checks, a few postcards. A notebook with my mother's name on the flyleaf, the pages mostly blank. A large, unlabeled manila envelope. I tell myself I cannot go through all this stuff—not now—but I open the envelope, which contains my parents' divorce papers, letters between their attorneys, and the birth and death certificates for my brother and sister. It seems my mother has filed together the evidence of Sad Inevitable Events without a warning label.

Digging deeper, I discover photo albums and papers that had belonged to my grandmother. I find report cards from my mother's elementary school days and a scrapbook my grandmother had filled with programs from every concert I'd ever played. There are loads of photos, many with annotations in my grandmother's elegant old-school handwriting, and a file folder filled with copies of Nana's poems. I can picture her typing them on the tan IBM Selectric typewriter that had retired with her from city hall.

Sitting on the wood floor in my mother's considerably less cluttered den, I find myself laughing as the word *baggage* pops into my head. Nothing like a metaphor come to life.

Fionah comes into the room, sizes up the situation immediately. "You'll want to zip that right up after you clean it off. Sure you'll go through everything another time. Shall I put on a pot of tea?"

Tea is in the kitchen and comes with sweets. Egg-eating Fionah eats no toast or home fries with her hearty breakfast omelets. She saves up her carbohydrate allowance to splurge on dark chocolate. "She's one of us," Tina had said when I mentioned Fionah's fondness for the dark stuff.

"We're nearly ready to paint," I say, a bit of optimism restored by the taste of 73 percent cacao.

"The house feels better already, Kate. Sure your mother has lovely taste, and I mean no offense. But going through her things with you makes me want to throw all my things away. I wouldn't want my Maureen to have to do this."

I'm not the fan of stuff that my mother is. Still, I have plenty of it. I consider my notable lack of offspring. Who would make the decisions to keep or to toss if I were to die an untimely death or drift into dementia?

"Will you do me a favor?" I ask Tina that night when we speak on the phone. "If you think I'm starting to show signs of Alzheimer's, would you suggest we clear the basement?"

"I'll help clear your basement if you help me with mine," she says.

Tina's promise makes me feel a little better the next day, when I scrub the suitcase with OxiClean, reload the contents, and move it into my mother's bedroom closet. Fionah is right— *another time.*

I will revisit that suitcase and its contents; photos and papers will be sorted into separate plastic bins, suitable for storage in my basement. Eventually I will toss the suitcase—nothing else. I will become the guardian for two generations of mothers and their miscellany, personal and public. I will be unable to let go of these paper traces of my mother and my grandmother. I will not ditch my grandmother's photographs, or the envelope stuffed with Sad Inevitable Events, or even the script my mother had saved from her production of *One with the Flame*, all overwritten with her director's notes. I'll take comfort in the keeping, even as I realize there's a lot to be said for traveling light.

Fionah and I develop a routine—clearing and cleaning, painting and rearranging. While we work, we talk. We swap stories. We share our worries. We voice our complaints.

"A couple of people have said to me, 'Now you know what it's like to have a kid.' It makes me so mad! First of all, my mother is not a child, and I don't want to treat her like one—ever. And if my mother were a child, I'd be looking forward to her future— not dreading it. My mother will move backwards in time, in knowledge, awareness. People with kids—they are in charge of little bundles of potential. I mean, there has to be some joy in that, right? Where's the joy in this?"

Fionah waits only a moment before she dives in. "Sure having children is no guarantee of endless joy." She smiles. "Even now, my daughter Maureen is grown and on her own, but I still worry over her. That's the same for you and your mom. You feel like you have to watch over her. When you have that deep sense of responsibility for another person—well, for me it's physical, like I carry a weight. I feel it like a pull in my stomach."

"Yes! When I think about my mother—even for a passing moment—I feel that too. It's a heaviness I haven't felt before. Even when I'm not worrying, I'm worrying."

"That's what you have in common with your friends with children now. Or at least your Irish friends with children," she amends.

Talk of family leads us to talk about love and romance. Fionah claims she has never been head over heels, never-look-back in love.

"Never?" I ask her.

"Never," she confirms. "You have. I can tell."

"Yes," I admit. "But I'm living proof that kind of love doesn't always mean a happy ending."

"Don't you know, marriage isn't the happy ending for the most of us." Fionah laughs. She presses me for details, which over the span of days and weeks I provide. When I come to understand that she has a crush on someone she's met recently, I encourage the romance, but she is hesitant to move forward. "Kate, I've slept with two men in my life, and I married the both of them. Please God, I don't want to make that mistake again."

"You don't have to sleep with him. Just kiss him," I suggest. We laugh as Fionah pours me another cup of red tea.

As much as we talk about love, we spend more time discussing death. "It's an Irish thing," she tells me. "We're obsessed with death and afterlife."

"I've never identified with being Irish," I've said to Fionah more than once.

"Look at your mother—look at your grandmother."

She laughs and tells me I can't help myself; I'm Irish. But those hyperproud Irish Americans bug the hell out of me, and the shamrock-and-green-beer Irish make me want to claim another nationality altogether. But who knows? Spending time with Fionah may rehabilitate me, restore in me some ancient Celtic pride.

"As a society, we're particularly unskilled when it comes to talking about death," Fionah says now. "For the Celts—and the Orthodox Jewish tradition is similar—mourning lasts a year and a day."

"I don't think it's only cultural, but historical too. As we become more 'modern,' we have less time for grief and grieving persons. You get a couple of days off work—and only if the death is in the immediate family—and you might get some special consideration for a couple of weeks. By then everyone has moved on—except the person or family who lost a loved one."

"And they feel this great pressure to get on with it, to act normal, when they don't feel normal at all." Fionah agrees. "We need to find a way to give people the space to grieve without feeling guilty or awkward."

"Or unproductive," I add, thinking how I felt pressured, after Eric died, to get back to work, to make sure those bookstores opened on time. Commerce does not stop for Death.

"You should write about it," Fionah says as our conversation moves into a familiar realm—my work as a writer, Fionah's work as a musician and composer. She's been researching the musical rituals around birth and death and has suggested we might create a book-and-CD package.

"Artistically, I'm more interested in the losses we suffer that are not physical death. As badly as we deal with the grief that accompanies death, I think we have an even harder time when we feel that same world-changing sense of loss when everybody is still alive."

"Are you thinking of your mum?"

"I wasn't, no. I was thinking about that novel of mine. The protagonist is unhinged by the voluntary departure of the man she loved. She can't get over him. And no one gets it, really—even she doesn't understand why she feels so bereft.

"But you might be right—about me thinking about my mom, I mean. Not just the Alzheimer's. That's the most recent loss, sure, and ongoing. But maybe because I've lost her before—to her work, to her marital difficulties, to her drinking—I guess I have no lack of material there."

Fionah smiles and gracefully changes the subject. "The place is looking good."

It is. With the help of my friend and Bog Boy, Tony, we've colored the walls in a palette of sun, sand, sky. The living room is a warm taupe; the kitchen is straw yellow with a blue door. The den is the same pale blue with gray-green overtones. The yellow from the kitchen lights up the hallway leading to the sunset rooms—the bathroom in an apricot-peach and the bedroom in a deeper orange-peach called Clementine. The trim throughout is a creamy white called Coconut Milk.

"The bedroom is brilliant!" Fionah says. "I love waking up in that warm orange—and those bright yellow doors." The closet doors were a risk, but the accent of bold golden yellow works with the orange, the creamy white, and the hammered black finish we sprayed onto all the doorknobs in the house.

"There are folks who won't think they want an orange bedroom, but I guarantee this house won't fade away in their memories," I reply. "Their realtor will show them a slew of tiny ranches, but this will be the one with the orange bedroom. They'll remember it. Color memory. That's my secret agenda."

"Sure your man Al won't forget it." Fionah laughs. In his real estate role, Al had stopped by while we were painting the bedroom. Wet on the walls, Clementine looked more like blood orange. Al seemed alarmed when he walked into the room.

"It will look amazing when it dries," I assured him.

"The rest of the place looks great," he replied. I thought he was reassuring himself. "Seriously, Kate. You've transformed this house. How soon can I start showing it again?"

"Next week," I told him.

There will be a few showings this month and next, and two offers. The first will be way too low and easy to decline; the second, contingent on a quick cash sale, will be withdrawn before we can come to terms. The weather will warm, the trees will leaf out, and then my mother's house—clean, clear, and colorful—will sell. It will sell in the spring.

Chapter Fifteen

In the Pink

My mother is moving down the hall, and her new room will be pink—Crayola Carnation Bubble-Yum Dum-Dum Bubble Gum Pink.

"What do you think, Katie?" my mother asks, pulling out a chip.

"I think it is definitely pink."

"Do you think it will be too much?"

"Well . . . if we go with a lighter tone, it will look too pastel."

"Oh, I hate pastels."

"Maybe something closer to coral?" I show her something less pink.

"How about that for the bathroom?" she asks.

"And the pink for the main room?"

"Yes. What do you think, Katie?"

"I think that when we first see it, we'll be surprised. But once we get your furniture moved in, and your pictures hung on the walls, it will be pretty, and bright."

"That's what I want: bright."

Bright enough that Mike, Sunrise facilities manager and de facto painter, called me. "Before I put on a second coat," he suggests, "maybe you should come take a look."

"Okay, but don't let my mother—or anyone else—in there before I see it." I work with colors a lot when I am doing book-store design work, and I have learned that folks often panic mid-paint job. Although the Sunrise leasing agreement specifically states that we can paint the walls whatever color we like—and we're paying for the privilege—I don't want any trouble about my mother's pinkening room until the paint job is complete.

When Mike unlocks the door, I can't help but giggle. Pink it is. It's not exactly Pepto-Bismol, but it is in the family.

"It's just the name—Peach Bloom—well, this doesn't look like peach to me, so I thought you ought to see."

"Maybe the color name comes from the flowers, not the fruit. This is the right color, for sure." I show him the chip. "It's powerful, but that's what she wanted. How's the bathroom?"

"Not so pink." He smiles. I step inside.

"This has more of the peach feel to it. I like it better, myself. But I think my mother will like the color of the main room. Do you mind if I get her?"

When she peers into the room, my mother starts laughing. "This is the color I picked?" she asks me. "Pink?"

"Yup, Mom. This is it." I hold the chip against the wall.

"Pink!" She whoops with laughter. I can't help joining her. Mike smiles, though I can tell he isn't sure how to interpret this outbreak.

"The walls glow in the afternoon light," I say when I regain my composure. "It feels warm and happy."

"And pink!" she says gleefully. "Nobody else in this place has a pink room!"

∽

The path to the pink room has been crooked and circular. Al-most everything about my mother's illness, I am learning, has a circular quality to it. Forgetting, reminding, remembering, forgetting. I experience the circularity not only in conversations with my mother now, but also in her actions and reactions, her moods, and her manner. When I visit, she is at first happy to see me. She likes to show me off to her friends. "This is my daughter," she says. My presence elevates her status among the ladies whose daughters are not in evidence. While we run errands or go shopping, she is content, though she tires quickly and cannot bear weight on her hip for long. Over dinner she often complains about her living situation, but I can usually redirect the conversation to more pleasant topics. But in the car on the way back to Sunrise, she grows angry with me. "You can't imagine what it's like living at that place!"

Sometimes my mother warms again before we say our goodbyes. Sometimes she does not. Either way, I leave Sunrise feeling worn down, sad, inadequate, and exhausted.

"I know I can't expect appreciation, but it would be nice to feel like my mother isn't eternally mad at me."

Suzanne reminds me of something we've discussed before. "Alzheimer's patients are constantly frustrated. And afraid. In the stage that your mother is in, it's not uncommon for the patient to blame everything and everybody around her for all the things that just don't make sense anymore. If your mother admitted the trouble was with her own mind—even if she could figure that out or remember it was true—it would be way too scary. So she makes it your fault. You are like the lightning rod for your mother's anger. And there's also a lot of history between you. That influences how she acts and how she feels around you. And how you act and feel too."

"Even if she can't remember the history?"

"She's not there yet, where it is all gone—she may not be able to remember or articulate specific details, but she still feels it."

"And I can remember the details. You're saying, for example, that my mother's habit of telling you that I'm wonderful and telling me I suck activates old issues for me."

"Does it?"

"Yes," I admit. "The feelings are familiar."

"Think of it a different way. You have always been the one constant in your mother's life. She loves you, and she knows you love her. When you're there, she feels safe—safe enough to be angry."

༄

I always feel better after I speak with Suzanne. She spends half an hour a week visiting with my mother and a second half hour following up with me by phone or by e-mail. If more time is required—and so far, it seems like more time is always required—Suzanne is flexible. I am paying the bill for her services out of my mother's account, but Jack has told me he's willing to subsidize this expense too, until my mother's house sells. I'm grateful for Jack's offer of backup funds. I'd be lost without Suzanne's support, which is not only psychological but often practical.

Only a few weeks after my mom moved into Sunrise, I got a call from Laurie, the residential supervisor. "We need to discuss some concerns we have regarding your mother. Recently the television remote went missing from the lobby, and it was found in your mother's room."

"My guess would be that she thought it was a telephone. She had that problem at my house sometimes."

"Perhaps, but we've also found a couple of knickknacks in her room. Nothing of value, but they aren't hers."

Personality changes accompany Alzheimer's, to be sure, but I couldn't imagine my mother turning into a late-life criminal.

"Well—umm—she's still adjusting to living there, and she may get confused about which is her room, what belongs to her—that sort of thing."

"Yes, I agree, and we do have residents who have similar behaviors. We can keep a watch on it. What we really need to talk about are the cigarette butts we've found in her wastebasket."

I allow myself a moment to reflect on the invasiveness of checking the contents of somebody's trash before I jump to my mother's defense.

"She's not smoking in her room. I'm supersensitive to cigarette smoke. I visit two or three times a week, and I would notice it. Here's the thing. When my mother stays at my house, I make her smoke outside. There's an ashtray next to a bench in the front yard, but sometimes she likes to sit on the deck instead. When she comes back inside, she carries in her dead butt and tosses it into the kitchen trash. She's probably doing the same thing at Sunrise."

"That's what she said she was doing."

"You've already spoken to her about this?"

"About the smoking, yes. She got very angry—almost aggressive—when I brought it up."

"Well, I believe she told you the truth."

"But even if she's only smoking outside, we can't have her putting cigarette butts into her coat pocket and carrying them into the building. What if one isn't all the way out? It's a real safety hazard. I told your mother that if she didn't use the ashtray outside, we would have to view her smoking as a supervised activity."

I couldn't imagine how much extra we'd be charged for the privilege of this particular supervised activity. Would they charge by the day or by the cigarette? I knew Laurie was doing her job, and I supposed it was possible that at some point

in the future my mother might carry an unextinguished cigarette in her parka pocket. But right now she was doing her best
to follow the rules. She was smoking outdoors, even in cold
weather, and she was being careful not to leave any butts on the
lawn. As I pictured my mother enjoying her cigarette, I realized
we were dealing not with a behavior issue but with a logistical
problem.

"My mother likes the sun. She usually sits at one of the
tables by the gazebo. The only reason she would carry her butts
inside is because there isn't a nearby ashtray. If we can place one
where she sits, I think that might solve this problem."

"I'll look into it," Laurie said, without enthusiasm.

Suzanne, when I called her a few minutes later, was happy
to follow up. "I'm also certain that your mom isn't smoking in
her room. I know where she sits when she smokes, and you're
right: there are no ashtrays in that area. I'll work this out with
Laurie. Don't worry, Kate. Your mother won't be kicked out."
She chuckled.

Or ostracized as a thief? These were my real fears, and I
could express them to Suzanne. And even feel relieved when
she laughed at them.

"When you first have a parent in assisted living, it's a little
like having a kid in summer camp or boarding school. You want
them to fit in, to be liked. Everyone already loves your mother."

"Everybody except Laurie," I couldn't help saying.

"She's just doing her job. I promise it will be okay."

And it was okay, thanks largely to Suzanne's intervention.
She found out the missing knickknacks didn't belong to another
resident, but rather were decorations my mother had lifted from
a table in the hallway.

"Oh," I said, "I bet she's rearranging." I explained to
Suzanne how my mother loved finding just the right spot for

every object. "And she may be unclear about what belongs to her, with moving and all."

"That sounds right to me. Why don't you bring some of her Hummel figurines on your next trip? If your mother is surrounded by more familiar objects, I think she'll be better able to distinguish what is hers."

~

As much as I appreciate Suzanne's moral support, her understanding and knowing ways with me, what I like best about Suzanne is that she likes my mother. She is developing a relationship with a woman she calls Anne, a person who is not only my mother, not only a patient with diminished capacities, but a woman with a personality as large as life, a still-quick wit, and a hard-to-resist rebellious streak. When she speaks of my mother, Suzanne speaks with a growing fondness, a tenderness. At the same time, she remains matter-of-fact about my mother's memory loss and understands her limitations. And she isn't afraid to step into the fray.

"When Anne asks when you are bringing her car, just say it is still in the garage. Eventually she will forget and stop asking."

I followed Suzanne's instructions for several weeks, but my mother didn't forget about her car. She invoked instead her seemingly reverse capacity to cleave onto one thing—a fact, an incident, or a desire—and become obsessed with it. When I said the mechanic deemed her car undrivable, my mother insisted I bring it anyway. If it were in the parking lot at Sunrise, she told me, she could sit inside and have a smoke.

"Mom, I can't tow the car thirty-five or forty miles just to provide you with a heated smoking lounge!"

I'd read about the struggle over driving and not driving in

some of the books I'd been reading about aging and dementia. I realized that hoping my mother would just forget about her car wasn't going to work. I talked to Suzanne. "I think even more than her house, the car is a huge symbol of independence for my mother. And my mother's identity—not unlike my own—is built on the fact of her independence. She's given up so much already."

"For safety's sake," Suzanne clarified for me. "Anne isn't living on her own because it is no longer safe for her to do so. And it isn't safe for her to drive, either, or even sit in the car smoking." She chuckled. "Leave it to your mother to think of that one. Listen, Kate, I'll talk to her. I'll play the heavy. I'll tell your mom that I've made the determination that it's no longer safe for her to drive."

The following week Suzanne reported back to me. "She took it fairly well. Anne asked me if I honestly felt it wasn't safe for her to drive, and I repeated that I did. Then she just changed the subject. Now, there's no telling whether she will remember this conversation, and she may bother you about it when you talk to her or see her. But remind her what I said and just stick to your guns. And let me know if I need to repeat the conversation with her."

During my next visit with my mother, the car was not mentioned. "My damn computer is broken again," my mother said when she saw me. My mother complains of computer problems on almost every visit, and some portion of my time is usually spent troubleshooting. Often I can locate and solve the problem with relative ease. She has inadvertently disconnected the phone line: I reconnect, and she is back online. She has forgotten how to get online: I write down the steps in the notebook we bought, and then I ask her to follow the directions. She forgets again: I remind her she can check the notebook. She confuses the computer and the television set: I remind her that the remote isn't meant to work with her turquoise desktop computer, which I suggest she leave turned on with her e-mail program open. (Forget the forgotten notebook.)

Unable to uncover the source of the problem on this occasion, I made the dreaded telephone call to AOL.

"Yes, miss. We have suspended this account due to suspicious activity." The AOL representative spoke with an East Indian accent, and he delivered this news with utmost politeness.

"Suspicious activity?"

"Multiple e-mails originating from this account. We do this to protect our members from spammers."

"My mother is seventy years old, and she has lapses in memory. Sometimes she forgets she has already sent an e-mail and sends another. I can assure you that she is not spamming anyone!"

"You see, the first time we see activity, we flag the account. When it repeats, we take away the e-mail privileges."

"What kind of activity, exactly?"

"I see this account most recently sent three hundred simultaneous messages."

Three hundred messages, as it turned out, to herself. I have no idea how my mother did it. "Sometimes my fingers slip," she told me.

We're not going to bring the computer to the pink room down the hall. My plan is to leave the digital age behind and see if my mother notices. I haven't had an e-mail from her in some time; these days, her obsessions run toward the noises in the kitchen that wake her every morning and her borrowed single bed. When she stretches in her sleep, she claims, she bruises her hands on the hardwood headboard. The bruises on her shins are also the fault of the bed, though I am unclear exactly why.

But these are things I can fix. It looks like the house is going to sell this time. We'll be able to afford a new bed with a latex mattress and an upholstered frame in a room far from the kitchen and the early morning noises.

My mother's pink room creates quite a sensation, even before she moves into it. Her lady friends come check it out, and my mother monitors the progress on the second coat. If she isn't sure she likes the color, she is sure that she likes the idea of the color, the outrageousness of the color, the pleasant shock of it when she opens the door. "It's the only pink room in the whole building," she declares, and in her voice I hear something I can only call pride of place.

Chapter Sixteen

Imperfection

"He doesn't know his woodwinds from his outwinds."

My mother is talking about her brother, my uncle Jack.

"Is there any chance you could get Mom to my concert on the Cape?" I'd asked him a few weeks earlier. "She loves to come to the concerts, but Noelle isn't able to pick her up this time. I'll get her back to Sunrise afterwards. You can head straight home." I hated to impose, but I knew my uncle was planning to visit Mom that weekend. He agreed to deliver Mom to the concert, but told me he'd be able to stay for only a couple of numbers. He wanted to get back to Worcester before dark.

"That will be fine. She'll be okay once she's in the auditorium," I told him. "Just get her seated and oriented. I can check on her at intermission, and I'll see if I know anyone else who might be able to sit with her. But even on her own, Mom will be fine. The situation is familiar to her."

I was disappointed my uncle wouldn't be able to stay for the whole program. Jack, like most of my family members, has never heard me play in a concert setting. I welcomed an opportunity to justify my musical existence in his eyes and ears. Still, I felt edgy about his presence in the audience. He and my aunt Jane are classical music fans who attend a lot of concerts in and around Worcester. The band is the band. We put on a good show, but we aren't exactly highbrow.

Jack surprised me by sticking around. Taking this as a good sign, I asked him as we were leaving the auditorium, "Did you enjoy the concert?"

"Well, the second half was definitely better."

Funny, I'd thought we'd had a killer first half of the program and that we'd lost some concentration in the second half. But I said nothing.

"There was something not right in the woodwinds in the first half," he said. "And the lead clarinet player—well, we were sitting in front of his wife, and I overheard him during intermission tell her that something wasn't right. But the second half was much better."

"Well," I said—willing myself to smile, trying hard not to take personally Jack's assessment of the concert I'd just played—"we ain't the BSO."

I invoked the Boston Symphony Orchestra for the sake of—what? Humility? Peace? Jack had gone out of his way to get Mom to the concert, and that was the main thing. I thanked him. After goodbye hugs all around, Jack made his way to his car. My mother and I stood in the doorway for a moment as I found my balance—music stand in my left hand, flute bag over my left shoulder, and my right hand free to hold my mother's as we crossed the parking lot.

"Can you believe he said that?"

"Said what?" My mother had forgotten Jack's assessment of the concert.

"Instead of just saying yes, he enjoyed the concert, Jack launched into a critique."

"Tell me what he said."

Clicking my mother's seat belt into place, I obliged with a repeat of Jack's remarks.

"Jack!" she said, shaking her head. "He doesn't know his woodwinds from his outwinds."

"Mom—" I protested her uncharacteristic bathroom humor for a single syllable before we gave in to a fit of giggles.

A few minutes later she has forgotten her wit, forgotten her brother's judgment, forgotten everything but how much she loved the concert. I let her tell me—again and again—what a great concert it was. And just for fun, I tell her what she said about Jack.

"I said that?"

I give her a nod.

"Well, it's true. My brother Jack can be an old fart."

"Outwinds," I repeat, and as if on cue, we dissolve into giggles.

One more time.

The cycle of repetition has the capacity to make me crazy— and often it does. But I've discovered recently that when I relax into it—cycle and recycle—repeat, respond, repeat—I understand there is comfort in the repetition. I've learned, for example, that if my mother initiates the repeat conversation, she is truly interested in the subject or has something she wants me to know. Today I am learning that laughter is always worth repeating. As we eat our dinner and I get Mom resettled into her room, I become my mother: telling and retelling the same story, relishing the joy she experiences when she realizes how clever she still is. We laugh. And we laugh again.

∽

"If you can't say something nice," my mother taught me as a child, "don't say anything at all." She didn't mean it as a motto to live by, but more as a key to pleasant conversation, a lesson in tactfulness. She wanted me to understand that there are occasions in daily discourse when discretion is required, and times when you might have to stretch to find that "something nice" to say. I know my grandmother was the original subscriber to the "something nice" theory; surely my uncle has at least a passing familiarity with the concept.

Was there really something wrong in the woodwinds during the first half of the program? I can't say for sure. Possibly a flat note in a duet, maybe a shaky rhythm in the backup part. Nothing your average audience member would notice—or hang on to. Was it that difficult for Jack to find the "something nice" to say? Why the analysis of our performance? Why couldn't he sit back, let go, and enjoy the music?

Easier said than done.

The reason I'm troubled by Jack's critique: he reminds me of me. Here I am, two weeks after the concert, and I am still replaying it in my head, trying to hear what wasn't right and hoping to God that I didn't play a role in the alleged musical offense. In my life, in my work, and in my music making, I want to make everything right. And until I was about thirty, by right I meant perfect.

My perfectionist streak, I've learned, is one of the classic reactions of kids who grow up in chaotic homes. Could I blame my younger self for trying to make right whatever she could? But as most of us discover, that need to be perfectly in control doesn't always serve or protect.

Several years after I began playing with the band, our lead percussionist gave me a poster of a silver flute with some sheet music artfully arranged around it. In white lettering on a black background were the words "Practice Makes Perfect."

"It reminded me of you," Dave said to me. This is the same man who had told me, after a rehearsal of a piece in which I had an extended solo, "I'm in heaven when I hear you play."

Words I never forgot, because not a season later he passed away—the day after our Christmas concert. I was touched by Dave's thoughtfulness and certain that he meant the poster as a compliment. Still, I considered tossing it. Worried about the bad karma of such a disposal, I kept it, all rolled up and stashed in a corner of the kitchen. But the truth is—and it has taken me long years to come to this understanding—practice does not make perfect. And for this I am grateful. Because I have come to believe—along with the French philosopher Voltaire, who said it in 1764—"The perfect is the enemy of the good."

As band members, we do pursue good—even excellence—in our musical endeavors.

"Mark that for woodshedding," our conductor is fond of saying about a tricky technical passage. John means he wants the players to go home, work and rework, play and replay a section until they can play it well. Most of us, myself included, will do as he asks. In the weeks between first rehearsal and concert, we will work to get it right.

John asks us to practice, but he does not expect or even desire perfection. What he wants from the fifty musicians who await his downbeat is *music*. "I don't want to hear a note recital," he says at rehearsals when the band is playing well, but without intention or musicality. He means he wants us to feel the music—whatever the style—and to carry the feeling forward so the audience gets something besides the notes.

John once told me his favorite day with the band is the day of the concert. "That's when we have the most fun," he said. At the time I questioned his use of the word *we*. I don't know if it's possible to relax and have a good time as a performing instrumentalist in a concert band or an orchestra. My experience is that the times are more fun in rehearsal, or when I'm playing jazz tunes with Harry or Egyptian pop with the four other members of our Arabic band. I suspect it's a little easier to have musical fun when there aren't forty-seven other people involved, each caught up in making sure to do the right thing, play the right note at the right time with the right level of intensity. There's too much interdependency. One reason I worry about my part so much is I know that my blowing a single line can lead to another player's confusion. The trickle-out effect of one mistake is nothing less than stunning in a group like ours.

"Oh, if somebody blows a section or a solo," John said to me a couple of years ago, "that's okay. Like at that concert where the baritones took off like a house of fire—and later, when the trombones weren't playing on the downbeat."

Oh, that's what happened, I thought to myself, remembering those several moments of thinking, *What the hell?*

"But it got itself together."

I noticed how John used the word *it*—referring to the music, rather than the band or even the conductor. He didn't say, "I had to work like hell to get us back together." He didn't say, "The band pulled itself together." *It got itself together.* John believes in the music, and in the power the music exerts over musicians—all of us, on and off the podium. The music, and our understanding of it, will get us through those scary moments. The music will assert—and reassert—itself. And what's interesting, too, is that John doesn't focus—the way I would if I'd been the player missing the downbeat or rushing past the beat altogether—on what went wrong. He notices it and moves on.

"Overall," he said, "that concert was one of our better performances."

Overall, I thought, but did not say aloud, is the key word in that sentence.

At the concert two weeks ago, the baritones did not take off like a house of fire. The trombones did not play the downbeat on the upbeat. And if there was "something not right in the woodwinds" during the first half of the program, I am pretty sure it was nothing that would ruin the music itself.

〜

"When is your next concert, Katie?" my mother asks me. We're on our way out for ice cream.

"Not till the fall," I tell her. "We don't play in the summertime."

"Oh, I wish you did. That was such a great concert."

I know she doesn't remember the music in any specific way, but she remembers something. Maybe a feeling that she associates with going to concerts. A feeling of *feeling-good*.

"When is your next concert?" she will ask me for several more months, until I can say "In a couple of weeks." Then I will tell her something about the program, something that might interest her. She will listen—carefully—and even ask some questions. And a couple of minutes later, she will ask me, "When is your next concert, Katie?"

I don't mind. I see now that the concert matters to her, that the music matters, and that my making the music matters to her even more. She does not require a perfect performance.

"Nothing in nature is perfect," I remember my mother telling me when I was seven or eight years old. As she pointed out the uneven structure, the lack of symmetry, the bumps and ridges in trees and flowers and seashells and rocks, she seemed to be telling me something about life. "Not perfect," she explained, "but still beautiful."

Why, I wonder, are we humans more comfortable pursuing perfection than accepting our natural, imperfect state?

We are sitting on stools in a small ice cream shop with a

view of Plymouth Harbor. My mother is eating a hot fudge sundae: coffee ice cream, hot fudge, and marshmallow topping. I'm sipping a raspberry-lime rickey.

"Yum," she says.

"Is it good?" I ask by way of making conversation.

"Delicious," she affirms.

In a perfect world, my mother would not be living at Sunrise. She would be living at home with me, and I would have the time, the skill, the financial stability, and the unceasing patience to care for her. But wait—in a perfect world, my mother would not have Alzheimer's. She would be living on her own, and we would meet for Indian-food lunches and go shopping together.

This is not a perfect world.

And this moment: it is a perfectly imperfect moment.

Aiming for perfection is easy, really. Accepting imperfection, I've discovered, is a much tougher proposition. I've learned this from music. I've learned this from life. And I've learned this from my mother.

"Yum," my mother says again.

"It's good," I say.

"Delicious."

Chapter Seventeen

Bad News Santa

A hospital emergency room is possibly the worst place on earth to have a panic attack. First of all, you're surrounded by medical personnel, one of whom might notice you. And ask whether you are okay. When you can't answer, she might do something crazy like take your pulse. The next thing you know, you'll be hooked up to an EKG, with a nurse preparing an IV drip, and your mother—your poor, frightened, and unwell mother—will be asking, "Where is my daughter?"

We've been in the ER since a little after ten in the morning. It is now nearing five o'clock in the afternoon. My mother is hooked up to various machines that are monitoring her heart-beat, her blood pressure, her blood oxygen levels. They have drawn her blood, taken a chest x-ray, and run an EKG.

The doctor is a good-looking, pleasant man whose first name, Scott, is engraved in blue on his white hospital badge, along with his surname and MD suffix. He tells me that the usual protocol would be to keep my mother overnight. "As I think Dr. Limbert explained to you, heart trouble in women, especially older women, doesn't always present with what we think of as the classic symptoms."

Dr. Limbert had told me exactly that when I reached her this morning. A little before nine, I'd gotten a call from the nurse at Sunrise. "Anne's blood pressure is quite elevated this morning, and she reports pain in the back flank area. Dr. Limbert wants her to go to the hospital."

Back flank area? I'm not even sure where that is. I looked at the clock, ran some quick calculations that did not include taking a shower. "I can be there in fifty minutes, tops. I can take her in, unless you think she needs to go sooner."

"No, that should be fine. We'll keep an eye on her in the meantime."

I was relieved that my mother wouldn't have to travel to the hospital in an ambulance. "This isn't a healthy place," she has said about Sunrise. "I've never seen so many ambulances. They come and go at all hours."

Early on, I had interpreted my mother's comments as another expression of her dissatisfaction with her new residence. It took me a couple of months to realize she was truly unnerved by the sight of an ambulance parked in the circular drive. It took me a couple more months to understand that their routine arrivals and departures were enough to unsettle me too. And I was a visitor. What must it be like to be living there, knowing one of your neighbors is being wheeled into an emergency vehicle? Wondering if you might be next. Nothing like mortality staring you in the face, flashing its red and white lights through the picture window of your new pink room. I couldn't imagine how terrified my mother would have been had she been loaded into an ambulance rather than coaxed into my passenger seat all those hours ago.

But I really shouldn't be thinking of ambulances or mortality, specifically my mother's, at this moment in the ER. I need to maintain cool, calm, and collectedness. I need to reassure my mother that all will be well.

"I'm not staying here overnight," she has declared at least

two dozen times. Her reasoning, also repeated: "People who go into the hospital never come out."

"The doctor may want you to stay, just tonight, for observation," I made the mistake of saying earlier this afternoon.

"I will refuse. I am not staying here overnight. People who go into the hospital never come out."

"Mom—"

"I am not staying here overnight! They can't keep me here if I refuse."

In fact, they can. So long as I approve. Since the day—right around this time last year—when my mother asked the attorney to sue me, I have been my mother's health care proxy. I choose not to remind her of that.

"Okay, fine, let's just wait to hear about the tests, okay? Can I get you some yogurt or something from the cafeteria?" "I'm starving," she says. "How about dinner?"

"Let me see what I can find." In the bustle and confusion of the morning, we have both missed breakfast. We've been here through lunch. It's now nearing dinnertime, and my blood sugar has crashed. I am shaky and primed for the anxiety attack I've been fending off for hours. Maybe a trip to the cafeteria will help—a few minutes away from the buzzers and alarms, the gurneys and the fast-moving medical personnel in their squishy shoes. I don't want my mother to realize I am not the even, reliable daughter I've been all my life—until this summer.

In May, my mother's house sold. Fionah helped me through one final round of clearing. Some of my mother's things we were able to sell; some we had hauled away; some we boxed for future review and moved into my basement. My mother—aware of the sale, though not present for the passing of papers—settled into her new pink room at Sunrise. She seemed, if not happy to be there, socially engaged and content. Our visits were easier; she was pleased to see me, no longer as steadfastly angry with me. In July, when my mother's Medicare coverage was finally reinstated, we followed up on Suzanne's referral to a smart, kind, and respectful geriatric specialist, Dr. Limbert. She comes to Sunrise to see my mother at least once a month and talks to me regularly by telephone.

With the sale of the house, my mother's financial transactions were less complicated for me to oversee. I paid Jack everything we'd owed him and put enough money into the joint account to cover the next several months of my mother's expenses. The rest I stashed in CDs with a series of maturity dates based on my calculations of how much money we would need and when. The monthly bills were now relatively predictable: rent, cable, my mother's medications, her telephone bill, the all-important quarterly Medicare premium, the copayment for the rented oxygen machine that Dr. Limbert had prescribed.

I felt like things were falling into place, that my mother and I had come to some sort of stasis, a place, I knew, not of perfection but of manageability. But my nervous system had its own agenda. When I experienced my first panic attack, I was with Fionah, sharing an Indian dinner. We were eating and chatting, and all was well. She was telling me a funny story when I felt this overwhelming, deeply physical dread. I found I couldn't focus on what she was saying. It was as if her voice were in the next room. Or more accurately, I had moved into another room. I had a hard time getting a deep breath, yet I wasn't wheezing. I felt like there was a volcano in my stomach. Because I had never before experienced something like this, I wasn't sure what was happening. I took a hit off my inhaler. I went to the bathroom. I said nothing to Fionah, but rather tried to focus on her words, which, due to the buzzing in my brain, were essentially unintelligible.

"I don't feel well all of a sudden," I managed at last. "Do you mind if I leave you some cash and go?"

I made it home, where I felt almost okay for a couple of hours. But the inexplicable array of symptoms returned just after midnight. I blamed the intestinal symptoms on the heaviness of the lamb dish we'd shared, my edginess on the caffeine in the spiced tea. The humidity was at fault for the tightness in my chest. The tingling limbs and unrelenting fear? I figured it was a combination of all of the above, exacerbated by the silent dead of the night. I considered calling 911, but the thought of trying to explain what was happening to me seemed more frightening than what I was experiencing.

The first episode seemed to last an eternity. Even when the intensity decreased, I remained anxious and wakeful till dawn. A week or so later, I had another—again without warning, this time in daylight. I did some research and confirmed that I was experiencing classic panic attacks.

I wasn't willing to share that with the world—not only because I felt embarrassed, but because even talking about anxiety can make you feel anxious. But I told Tina what was happening, and I was surprised to hear that she had her own experiences with anxiety. So did Suzanne, who suggested, among other things, that I change the radio station if I feel an attack coming on while I am driving. "Do any small thing that makes you feel like you have control."

I felt comforted to learn that people I knew had experienced this level of anxiety. Tina told me I could call her anytime I felt the panic rising. "Sometimes it just helps if you can hear another voice besides the one inside your head that is making you freak out."

My friend Harry—kind, empathic, with an ever-mordant wit—told me, "To be honest, Kate, I'm just surprised that it's taken you this long to feel anxious." The panic, and especially its timing, may be irrational, he seemed to be saying, but the ongoing stress in my life—that is real.

Anyone who experiences anxiety attacks will tell you that the worst thing about them is you never know when you might have another. This creates a free-floating, nonspecific nervousness in between full-blown episodes. As summer turned to fall, I sought help from homeopathy and acupuncture, but I also found myself rearranging my life to accommodate the anxiety. A panic attack at my busy hairdresser's sent me home without the cut—though I did manage to stay there until it was time to rinse the color. I changed stylists so I could make my appointments when the salon was nearly empty. I had another episode at a restaurant; I avoided eating out. I found I couldn't visit Tina in New Hampshire—the drive, especially through the tunnels, terrified me. Even driving to Plymouth to see my mother was a challenge during what I now think of as my "peak anxiety" period.

When the third Monday in September rolled around, I wasn't sure I could make it through a band rehearsal. I remember sitting in my car, in the parking lot, gripped by a dread that was much deeper than my standard Monday night butterflies. I made it inside and was relieved to see that the music was not demanding—no big solos, nothing to make me even more anxious than I already was. The time spent playing proved to be time free from panic. Of course, living through the rests and interacting with my fellow band members on breaks was another matter entirely. Every practice session was a challenge, but in meeting that challenge every Monday night, I grew more confident in my ability to live through and move past the anxiety.

Out of my mother's line of sight, I shake five of the round homeopathic pellets out of the little amber bottle I carry in my purse and pop them under my tongue. I breathe to prove to my asthmatic self I am fine. I *will* be fine. The panic isn't here yet; it is only hovering. What else can I do to fend it off? Oh, right—go to the cafeteria. Maybe getting food is a way to exert control. Will I be able to manage if it's crowded?

Before I can decide, I feel a hand on my shoulder. It's the ER doctor with a sheaf of paperwork in his hand.

"I've got some results now," he says, "and I spoke to your mother's doctor. Given your mother's . . . mental situation, it's probably best we speak alone for a minute. The chest x-rays show a couple of spots on your mother's left lung. We'd need a CT scan to see what they are. But to be honest with you, given your mother's history—breast cancer, smoking—there's a pretty good chance we're looking at malignant tumors."

All I can think to say is, "Okay."

"Dr. Limbert isn't too concerned about heart issues right now. The EKG showed some abnormalities, but the results weren't inconsistent with past testing. The spots on your mother's lungs provide a possible explanation for the pain she reported this morning. That pain may have caused her blood pressure to rise. It's within normal range now. I know she doesn't want to stay here tonight, and I don't feel, given this information, that I need to keep her in the hospital."

"Well, she'll be glad to hear that. As for the other—I don't know how much she will be able to take in or process. Sometimes she clings to just one thing, even when she forgets everything else. I don't think we want that one thing to be the worry that she may have lung cancer."

"I understand. How about I mention we saw some spots on the chest x-ray and let her know she needs to follow up next week with her primary care physician?"

"Sounds good," I say, though I'm not sure anything sounds

good right now. As I consider the possibility—likelihood—that the spots on my mother's lungs are cancerous tumors, I also consider that my mother's decreased kidney function means she isn't a candidate for chemotherapy. Her asthma turned emphysema complicates her relationship with anesthesia, and I know that anesthesia and Alzheimer's is another bad combination.

"Dr. Limbert filled me in on your mother's other health issues," he says, as if he is reading my mind. "You'll have decisions to make about how you want to follow up. Dr. Limbert will help you. She said to tell you that you could call her anytime. But right now, I'll fill out the discharge papers so you and your mother can have Christmas."

∽

Merry Christmas.

I'd planned to grocery shop this morning, then pick up my mother and bring her back to my house. We'd have a big Christmas Eve dinner, open presents. I'd make brunch on Christmas morning and get my mother back to Sunrise before dark. But by the time we leave the hospital, all the stores are closed. There will be no food shopping today. Even our old standby, the Ninety Nine Restaurant, is already closed for the holiday. Back at my mother's room, I collect a few things for her visit. It will be the first time she's been back to my place since she moved into Sunrise. Until the bigger news of this day, I'd been worried about how the overnight would go. Now I'm just concerned that she gets in a session on her oxygen machine before we leave for the Cape.

"The road is so dark," my mother says on the way to my house. This statement braids with "I never knew you lived so far away" in the thought-speak-and-repeat cycle that accompanies our drive. She's already forgotten about the spots on her lung. "What a waste of time," she said as we pulled out of the hospital parking lot. "All that time waiting, and there's nothing wrong with me."

I see no reason to correct her revised version of our day. But I feel strange, and heavy, as I think about what I know about my mother that she doesn't know herself, medical truths she will never internalize, even if they are spoken aloud to her. *You have Alzheimer's. You may have lung cancer.* Do I owe her the truth, even for a moment? Or do I owe her tranquility, peace of heart—for as many moments, remembered and unremembered, as she has on this planet?

I find a parking spot right in front of the Chinese restaurant. It's eight thirty on Christmas Eve, and the place is hopping. There is a single booth open, and we slide in.

"What do I like, Katie?" my mother asks me, flipping through the menu.

"You like pork egg foo yung with lobster sauce," I tell her.

I look around the restaurant. It's filled with families— crammed into booths, in circles around large tables. The atmosphere is festive. I realize I have a choice: spots or no spots, a Christmas ruined or a Christmas to be treasured. I go for no spots. Not tonight. And maybe not tomorrow either.

"Merry Christmas, Mom," I say, raising the ivory porcelain teacup in a toast.

My mother lifts her teacup, touches mine. "Merry Christmas, daughter," she replies.

We sip strong black jasmine tea and wait for our food to arrive.

Chapter Eighteen

Hollywood Ending

For Christmas dinner, we eat leftover Chinese food. My mother, having no recollection of Christmas Eve, is surprised by the unusual holiday menu. I remind her where we were the day before, explain that I'd been unable to shop.

"Oh—right. Such a waste of time! All those tests just to find out I'm fine." She shakes her head before she digs into her reheated egg foo yung. I keep my own counsel across the table over my plate of Tofu Family Style, wishing I'd gone grocery shopping earlier in the week. I like to make a feast for holidays—and even more, I enjoy serving a complicated meal to a tableful of friends and family. My mother, Bruce, and Tina are the regular attendees, but we welcome drop-ins. Last year we hosted a small crowd of visitors on Christmas afternoon for the fig-laden medieval desserts that Bruce had helped me make. I'm in the early stages of a new book project set in the ninth century; the cooking and the serving were a convenient extension of my research.

This year Bruce is occupied with a new job in Vermont, and Tina had to work a London trip, returning on the twenty-seventh. On Christmas Day, it is just my mother and me and food that tasted better the night before.

We opened presents this morning. I gave my mother a

framed picture of Bix waking from a nap. He has a cold-weather habit of sleeping under the covers, head sticking out human-style. In the photo he is poised between waking and sleeping, eyes half-open, one paw stretching toward the camera. I'd sent the image as my holiday card this year. "Whenever I feel the least bit sad, I am going to look at that picture of Bix on my fridge and cheer up right away," Tina told me. I was hoping the image might inspire the same response from my mother.

"My grandchild," she joked when she looked at the photo. "You have a good life, don't you?" she said to Bix, who was curled up next to her on the couch. Then she opened her big gift: a warm but lightweight parka for her outdoor smoking ex-peditions. It's made of soft, silvery fleece, with fake fur trimming the hood and reindeer prancing across the hem. "It's so soft," she said, patting her new jacket like it was another kitty.

My mother surprised me with a creamy white scarf wrapped in a gift bag. I teared up when I realized that Suzanne must have taken her shopping. "I love it," I told my mother, "and I will get a lot of use out of it."

In midafternoon we make our way back to Sunrise in a heavy, crazy, no-visibility rain. I am tense with the driving, but intent on getting my mother back to her oxygen machine. Given the Christmas Eve discovery, I don't want her to miss any more treatments.

"Turn around, Katie. This rain is too dangerous. I'll stay at your place tonight."

"No, Mom. You're supposed to breathe twice a day on your machine, and you missed this morning and yesterday morning too. I need to get you back to Sunrise today so you don't miss another treatment."

Her tone shifts as she moves from mother-worry over driv-ing conditions to mother-anger over living conditions. "You're the only kid in the family who has put her mother away," she declares, an edge in her voice. I feel like she is spitting on me.

"Mom, you know your living situation wasn't safe anymore."

"Rosemary lives alone, and nobody's talking about putting her away."

"Rosemary doesn't have the same health issues you do— and she is six years younger. At some point she may decide she needs some assistance too."

"What about Jack? He's older than me!" Before I can respond, she answers her own question. "Oh, he has Jane. A *wife*. If I had a wife, I wouldn't have to live in this place."

"Mom—"

"Katie, you should be ashamed of yourself. You have taken the path of least resistance."

"No, Mom, I've taken the path to keep you safe. You know it wouldn't work out if you were to live with me—you'd be alone when I traveled, and face it, Mom, you need more support than I can give you. And at Sunrise, you have friends—"

"Bullshit. I live with strangers! You don't know how much I resent that! Rosemary doesn't have to live with strangers. Jack has a wife. I'm the only one."

Comparing her living situation with her brother's and sister's is a new variation on an old theme—one I thought we retired several months ago. But here we are—back to square zero, all good feelings vanished. She cycles and recycles. I count ten repetitions—almost word-for-word. I keep my cool, play my role in this emotionally fraught call-and-response. In an effort at distance, I consider the way my mother can still string the words together so well—*the path of least resistance*—and yet have no awareness she is repeating herself. Alzheimer's patients tend to lose vocabulary as the disease progresses. My mother, thanks perhaps to a lifetime of reading and writing and teaching, still holds on to most of her words and invents new ones for those she has lost—even as her memory grows increasingly unreliable.

It is a long, long ride to Sunrise. Inside the lobby, we discover the power is out. Is this my punishment for rushing my mother back to her machine? There will be no breathing treatment without electricity. A staff member assures me that Sunrise is a priority setting on the electrical grid; power will be restored quickly. In the meantime, my mother shows off her new coat. "My daughter gave it to me," she says proudly, taking in the compliments before she pours herself a cup of coffee. Watching her chat with her lady friends, I feel better about being the only kid in the family who has put her mother away.

After about twenty minutes the lights come on, and I set my mother up on her breathing machine. I plug in the lights on the tiny Christmas tree we had placed in the window of her room. "It's so pretty, Katie," my mother says.

"I'm going to head home before dark," I say.

"Thank you for a wonderful Christmas. I love this." She pats the parka draped over her shoulders.

Her room will heat up quickly, and in the meantime she has her reindeer coat to keep her warm. She is breathing on her machine and enjoying her Christmas lights. Outside, the rain is letting up. The western sky is streaked with pink and yellow. As I turn the key in the ignition, I feel empty, but relieved. The storm has passed.

∽

Three or four years ago, I filled out one of those silly Internet quizzes. You share your answers with the person who sent the quiz to you, and send the questions and your answers along to another group of friends who may or may not do the same. The point of these quizzes is that you are supposed to learn surprising details about folks you think you know.

Name your favorite movie, I read. *Mary Poppins,* I typed. I saw it in the theater when I was sixish, and it made a big impression. Bigger, perhaps, because I'd seen so few movies since. My friends would be surprised—not that I named *Mary Poppins* as my favorite movie, but that I could name any movie at all. I could count the movies I'd seen in my whole life on my fingers and toes with a foot and a half left over. And there was no chance of my seeing a movie on TV. I'd left off watching television in my teens. I was known and accepted as an innocent and an ignorant in the realm of all things celluloid.

Then *Cottage for Sale* was purchased by a publisher, and there was talk of making it into a movie—or even a TV show! I realized that I needed to bone up, to fill this gaping hole in my cultural education. I had a little white TV/VCR combo that I'd purchased to watch the video Harry had made of the cottage move. It was just sitting in the den. Why not put it to some use?

I began my journey at my local video store, renting mostly romantic comedies. I favored those set in New York or Paris. In fact, for a Paris setting and the French language, I was even willing to forego the happy ending. I sought suggestions from friends for movies that were light and easy. I'm affected by visual images, and I readily suspend disbelief. I wanted to watch movies, not live with them for weeks on end.

On the long-distance advice of my college friend Mimi, I rented the first season of *Sex and the City*. I loved the girls, their troubled love lives, their amazing wardrobes, and the soft-focus, high-glamour version of single life in New York. For me, the heart of the show was neither sex nor shoes, but the bond that endures between women, the families we create from friends. I couldn't wait to watch another season.

Cottage for Sale never made it to the screen—big or small—but I continue to receive and return a steady stream of DVDs in those nifty red and white envelopes. I watch movies as a writer—I am in awe of what a good script can accomplish in the span of 105 minutes—and character-centered TV writing fascinates me too. But I also watch to forget about the life outside the screen. During times of stress—and even when I feel the upcreep of panic—I can be diverted by twists and complications I know will be resolved without my intervention.

Bix enjoys the Netflix membership too. He cuddles up against me on the couch in the little yellow room, keeps an eye on the action—until he falls belly-up and snoring, sound asleep. He wakes for his favorite part: the fun buzzing sound of the tray when it slides open for me to take out the DVD at the end of the night. Sometimes I repeat the open-and-close a few times just for his amusement—and mine.

What I seek in these most recent evening hours, the coldest and darkest days of the year, is to find my own Hollywood ending. I don't mean the one where the perfect man realizes I am the perfect woman and chases me across town, running stoplights to get to the airport to catch me before I wing my way to Paris. (I don't turn around; he comes with me, of course.) No, I mean the one where Dr. Limbert hasn't called to tell me the spots on my mother's lungs have all the characteristics of malignancy. In my Hollywood ending, my mother is not presumed to have lung cancer—or if she has it, she isn't too frail or too memory-challenged to undergo surgery. Hell, maybe some miraculous discovery is made and her Alzheimer's is reversed. Or maybe it's a time travel thing, and we can travel back in time to the point before my mother's mind and body began to fail, and we can rearrange her DNA so that—what—she lives, if not forever, at least with all her mind and body parts healthy and intact?

"There is no way to know, without exploratory surgery and a biopsy, whether we are dealing with a metastasis of breast cancer to the lungs or a new cancer that has originated in the lungs," Dr. Limbert explained when she called with the CT scan results. "With your mother's history, either is possible."

She spoke slowly, softly, leaving space for me to fill, expecting me to ask questions. I had none. I wasn't surprised by the news—but hearing this confirmation of the worst-case scenario, I realized how much I'd been hoping the spots would be harmless scar tissue, that they could be explained away without any reference to cancer.

"Usually I would refer a patient with these results to a surgeon, but I think we really need to think hard about what surgery would mean for your mother."

"I'm worried about surgery, because the anesthesia is likely to make her Alzheimer's worse. But I know from the breast cancer treatment that Mom isn't a chemotherapy candidate. Is radiation an option?"

"You're right: chemo is out of the question with Anne's renal issues. But if you like, I can refer you to an oncologist."

"Well, what do you recommend?"

"Kate, I can't say that I recommend surgery. Radiation would take a big toll on her too—and it would only be palliative without surgery. The tumors are tiny. Anne hasn't reported any pain since Christmas Eve. There's a good chance that incident wasn't even related. We caught this almost by accident. Lung cancer is generally slow-growing. If the cancer originates there, Anne's other health issues are liable to cause more trouble before these tumors do."

"If we rule out surgery, radiation, and chemo, what we're talking about is—no treatment?"

"It's entirely up to you. Remember, if you make the decision not to treat the cancer, we can still treat any pain or discomfort that your mother may have. Think about what you want to do. We'll talk again. Call me anytime. And talk to Suzanne too. This isn't an easy decision, I understand."

Straightforward. But not at all easy. To say *I am going to allow a probable cancer to grow in my mother's body.* What kind of health care proxy makes that decision? Or: *I am going to allow my mother to suffer the trauma of surgery and the likely and potentially permanent aftereffects of anesthesia.* Are these my only choices?

&

A few days later I follow up with Suzanne. "In your experience," I ask her, "is the post-anesthesia decline in Alzheimer's patients permanent?"

"As we've said, there is always a worsening of the condition. The patient sometimes recovers some of what was lost—after a few weeks or a month. But usually, yes, some of what is lost is lost forever. There's no predicting how much."

"If I choose surgery, am I also choosing to move my mom out of Sunrise? Or into the Alzheimer's wing?"

"Again, so much of this is unpredictable, but your mother will probably need more care, either on a temporary or permanent basis."

"And if surgery reveals the tumors are cancerous, what does that do for us, really? I guess they can remove them, but if she can't take chemo . . . And radiation—I don't know if that's a real option either."

"Did Anne have radiation for the breast cancer?"

"Yes, and it took a lot out of her. And that was five years ago—she was a lot stronger then."

"That's something to consider too, Kate. Even if an oncologist is willing to prescribe radiation treatment, do you want to put your mother through that?"

"If she can't handle radiation or chemo, and if the cancer is already elsewhere in her body—or the tumors grow back after surgery—I mean, we're right back where we started, except that my mother has progressed more quickly into a deeper dementia."

"You don't have to rush into a decision here. You can decide not to treat for now and then see how things proceed."

But there's something in me that feels l need to make this impossible choice sooner rather than later. I feel too—despite the reassurances of Dr. Limbert and Suzanne that I can change my mind—that my decision will be irrevocable. Inaction is an action.

I remember when, some months into my mother's stay at Sunrise, her friend Josie moved into the Alzheimer's cottage. "They put Josie in lockdown," my mother declared. Suzanne had given me advance warning about the move, so I was prepared, though sorry, for the development. Josie, sweet and batty and childlike, was my mother's closest friend at Sunrise. I arranged for Suzanne to take my mother to visit her, but Josie didn't recognize my mother. "Josie has been drugged!" my mother told me. "She was fine last week! Her mean brothers must have decided she needed to be locked up."

"Mom," I began. "Josie just needs a little more help now—"

"Shoot me first, Katie," my mother said before I could finish my sentence. "Shoot me *before* I need to be locked up."

When I relate this exchange to Suzanne, she chuckles. "I can hear Anne saying that."

"The thing is—I know it isn't much to go on—but somehow, her saying that—well, it makes me think that she would want me to keep her away from surgery, protect her from the trauma that would cause a more rapid progression of the Alzheimer's."

"You have a lot to go on, Kate," Suzanne tells me. "You've known your mother your whole life, and you have done everything you can do to keep her safe and comfortable. You've made the right choice at every step of the way, and you'll make the right choice for you and for your mother this time too."

A few days later, when I call Dr. Limbert to tell her that we won't treat the cancer, I'm sure it is the right decision. At the same time, I think I have made a horrible choice. In the few months since the holidays, my mother has been easier, sweeter with me. She gives and receives hugs, and our visits are filled with good feeling and good humor. She isn't angry with me any longer. She's erased large chunks of unpleasantness from her memory, revised and improved her life story.

On some days, I believe, she is happy. And on those days I am either more sure or less sure I've made the right choice on my mother's behalf. I'm opting, I hope, for quality of life while my mother is alive—whether weeks, months, or years. I only wish I didn't have to choose between quality and quantity.

∾

This Sunday afternoon concert isn't too demanding for me. From the stage I can see my mother, installed in her favorite seat: stage left, three rows from the back, aisle seat. "I have the best view of you from there," she has explained to me.

After the concert, we'll have dinner at the Ninety Nine Restaurant and I'll deliver my mother back to Sunrise. She will have a cigarette while I park the car, and then we'll go inside and visit a little longer. Before I leave, I will give my mother an extra long hug and remind her that I'll see her in just a few days.

Back at home, I'll fire up the teakettle, and Bix will watch with interest while I slip in a DVD.

It's a comedy sort of night.

Chapter Nineteen

The Moment

When she isn't playing piccolo, Aileen knits. Even during dress rehearsal, for which we do not dress but during which we do not stop for anything or anyone. "Concert conditions," John likes to say.

"You must have nerves of steel," I say to her after we finish playing the prelude to *Die Meistersinger.* Aileen, age seventy-nine, is the sturdy second flute and piccolo in the Cape Cod Community Orchestra. I'm guessing she's played for at least sixty-five years, and I know that for some of those years she played piccolo for the Cape Cod Symphony. She reminds me of that now.

"Playing only piccolo," she says, "I'd be staring at fifty-two measures' rest." The implication is that while she wasn't playing, she had to do *something.* "It's just straight stitching," she adds. "Nothing complicated."

In the few seconds before we embark on Handel's *Overture to the Royal Fireworks,* I allow how I can't knit any stitch at all, straight or crooked, but I don't have time to say what I am really thinking: Even if I could knit, I can't imagine doing anything but staring straight ahead and counting silently to myself on those stretches between entrances. Okay, maybe the occasional prayer.

I've decided, in the one and one-eighth rehearsal I've attended for this concert, that I am a rehearsal kind of woman. I like the process of coming to understand the music, hearing the other instruments, the melodies and countermelodies, the supporting bass line. Understanding, on a level that is not so easy to explain, how my part fits in. I'll be playing this Sunday's concert on two run-throughs. Part of me thinks I was insane to agree to do it. The other part of me is grooving on the challenge. It's that latter part of me—in music and in life—that routinely gets me in trouble.

Our band director, John, began conducting this group just a few years ago. He's been working to grow the orchestra, but I notice we're still light on some of the string parts. I mention this to Aileen on the break.

"We used to have more violins," Aileen tells me. "But they just disappeared one by one." She shrugs.

"Plenty of cellos, though," I remark. I haven't had a moment to count them, but I am pretty sure there are more cellos than violins. Curious. To Aileen, I venture, "Could it be that violinists begin so early and stop playing—"

"Yes, once they know they're not going to make it."

"But people actually take up the cello later in life. They like the sound of the instrument."

Aileen nods. She acts as though I may have a point. "Nobody takes up the violin in the middle of their life." She smiles. Is it my imagination, or do her hands keep moving, even while she is speaking, even while she is looking at me straight on, swapping theories of late-life string playing?

Violists, I count two. Both older gentlemen in their sixties. Or seventies?

"No string bass at all," I say to Aileen. "In fact, no bass, period. No tuba or baritone horns. We're a little heavy on the soprano winds."

"My husband used to play string bass with us," Aileen offers.

I say nothing, wondering whether her husband has passed away.

"But he can't play anymore," she says. *Alive*, I think, and almost breathe a sigh of relief on Aileen's behalf before the word *Alzheimer's* comes unbidden into my head. I conjure other reasons why he might not be able to play. Unceasing arthritis in his hands? Can't finger the strings? Bad circulation in his legs, unable to stand for long periods? Chronic tendonitis in his bowing arm?

I remember a conversation with Bob one night after band. "I always had this theory that playing music protects your brain from Alzheimer's, but then Al had to go and get it." He was talking about one of his fellow first clarinetists. Well into his eighties, Al always wailed on the big band and Dixieland tunes. Al's younger wife, Deb, plays clarinet too. Though Al had gone missing this year, Deb still showed up every week.

"Oh—I didn't know," I said to Bob. One thing about playing with older musicians is that folks do disappear.

"My fingers, you know, the arthritis in my hands. It frustrates me. I can't play quick passages the way I could when I was younger. But the idea that I couldn't remember what the notes are, or the fingerings, couldn't read music—"

Aging with an instrument is fraught with difficulty. You have the potential to mature as a player. Through the years of playing, your understanding grows and your musicality increases, but your technique can be diminished by changes in your physical body. Bob has figured out how to work around his uncooperative third finger; already I deal with the neck and shoulder issues not uncommon in flute players. What scares us both to death is the thought that we could lose the capacity to adapt, to read, to play.

At the end of tonight's rehearsal, Aileen points to her black metal music stand. "I have another one of these in my car, if you want to use it at the concert." I've been using a folding stand, and it is a kind offer.

"Oh, I have my own, just like yours. I just didn't bother to haul it out for the rehearsal. I'll bring it for the concert."

"Well, you're welcome to mine. It's always in the car."

I consider the phantom stand; no doubt it was her husband's. I graciously decline. Musicians, some of us, are almost as superstitious as baseball players. It's not that my stand is lucky, but it has history, mine, and it is predictable. It works. It does not wobble nor lean, and it has handy little rubber booties on the three metal feet so that it doesn't scratch the floor. The booties are only fifteen years old, but the stand I've had since high school. It was a graduation gift from my high school band director. It came with a big pink bow, which for many years I left attached, until the pink faded to gray and began to disintegrate. The bow reminded me of a time when I thought music was it for me—the beginning, the middle, the end. A time of promise, a time of some small triumph, a time when someone believed in me, encouraged me, nudged me, and ultimately sent me off to music school with a sturdy metal stand.

∽

On Sunday, with my trusty music stand in position, I exchange hellos with Aileen, relieved to see she hasn't brought her knitting. She projects calm and preparedness, two qualities I wish I could summon. Before a concert, my nerves express themselves with an acutely physical impact—after a predictable and thorough cleansing of my digestive system, I am left with leaden butterflies, tingly fingers, shaking legs, shallow breathing, and a dry mouth. These out-of-control physical sensations wreak havoc with my mental capacity and throw open the door for any small doubts or insecurities to grow large and threatening.

The only way to get through the performance is to play the music. At my best, my concentration is laser-like; the audience is elsewhere, as are all the issues in my life or in the larger world. It is me, my flute, the notes on the page, my sound and the sounds around me, the interplay of the ensemble, the signals from the conductor.

At my worst? Well, I lose focus and screw up.

The advantage of playing a concert on two rehearsals is that I have no choice today but to concentrate. I don't know the music well enough to allow my mind to wander. I count my rests as if my life is on the line. Still, the voice of doubt manages to outpsych me on an early solo line I share with the principal clarinet. I sailed right through it on my first read, but I'd messed it up in rehearsal on Wednesday, and here I am, blowing it in concert. But a moment later I reenter, playing with the confidence that comes from getting those two measures out of the way. I have so many beautiful parts to play in the next seventy-five minutes. I've come to understand that errors are inevitable. What matters is not that we make mistakes, but that we recover from them. We find our way back, and we keep on playing.

∽

My *Romper Room* theology is eclectic and inclusive, perhaps because I left the church of my origin when I learned that my newly divorced mother was no longer welcome there. It was the late 1960s, and divorced Catholics were subject to excommunication. The way I saw it, the church had abandoned my mother when she most needed the solace of her faith. If they wouldn't have her, I decided, they surely wouldn't have me.

I have never returned to Catholicism or found my place in any organized religion, and I am resistant when anyone insists there is just one way to locate God or Enlightenment or Happiness or Truth or whatever it is we humans seek. I might be accused of a Chinese restaurant form of spirituality, choosing one from column A and one from column B, but I work to understand the various paths we humans blaze en route to Something or Someone larger than we are, and I find relevance and meaning in the multiplicity rather than the one.

When I play music, I do my best to follow the Buddhist instruction to be mindful, hoping to locate the space they call emptiness. In performance, you must show up for every musical moment. You must be present; you must inhabit that note, that measure, that phrase. And then you must forget it and move on. It turns out that a focus on the present and a letting go of ego concerns are also helpful guidelines when caring for a loved one with Alzheimer's.

For my mother, what matters is the moment we are in. There is no memory of the moment before, and the moment to follow is not the future so much as the new present—the moment we will inhabit as soon as this moment passes. My mother, even as her disease has progressed, is able to be in the present. There's no certainty how long her awareness will last; the cycles and recycles of conversation have grown shorter in recent months. But what I've come to recognize is how little that matters.

Memory is overrated. What is important in my mother's life, and in the time that I spend with her, is that we have those moments. I can string them together into memory, and she cannot. But what I believe—what I have to believe—is that the quality of the moment matters, if only in that moment. She may not remember what we had for supper or what we talked about while we were waiting for the food to arrive. But she enjoys the meal; she revels in the conversation. She will eat the ice cream for dessert with unabashed enthusiasm. And the next day she will say to Suzanne, "I haven't seen Kate in weeks. She's off on a job in California."

This no longer bothers me. I no longer feel the need to prod my mother's memory, to remind her, to prove that I am a dutiful daughter. I've learned to live life with my mother her way, moment to moment. Of course, I still think and plan as best as I can for her future—and I feel compelled, still, to worry over it, especially late at night. But when I am with my mother, it's like I am with the music. I am there, present and attuned. Mindful of the moment now, and yet mindless as the moment, passing, becomes past.

Chapter Twenty

Mother's Day

Before I dial the phone, I consider the possible greetings. *Happy Soon-to-Be-a-Mother's Day*. That sounds like it is the holiday, not the motherhood, that is imminent. *Happy Soon-to-Be-a-Mother Day*. Is it okay to drop the possessive on *Mother*? *Happy Almost-a-Mother Day*? Better.

I hear Tina's melodic, upward-rising "Hello?"

"Happy Mother's Day," I say, ditching all the provisional stuff and going for the classic wish.

"Thanks. Jonathan gave me flowers."

"Oh, good, good. Next year he won't have time to do that. How do you feel?"

"Nauseous. The only thing that helps is to eat something, and that only helps temporarily. Till I eat something else. At this rate, I'll be huge by next week."

We laugh, and neither of us says what we are both thinking: the nausea is good. Tina miscarried last year, and the first sign of trouble was the sudden disappearance of her morning sickness—which in Tina's case should be more aptly called all-day-long sickness. The part of me that worries about what my mother calls "tempting Fate" hesitated about marking Mother's Day too soon; Tina is just rounding the bend of her first trimester. But I have this unwavering confidence that Tina and baby will be fine this time. It isn't merely hope. I feel certain of it. I'm also sure that Tina is having a girl.

"Eating is good," I pronounce. "Keep at it."

Tina knows me well enough to follow my unspoken train of thought. "How's your mom?" she asks.

"All I can say is, thank God for Boost. She drinks a bottle two or three times a day. She never gets up for breakfast anymore. She skips lunch most days, and she rarely eats anything at dinner. She still eats when I take her out, so it isn't like she has lost her appetite. I almost wonder if she forgets—you know—one moment she feels hunger, but before she acts on that, she's forgotten the feeling. Or maybe she has forgotten what the next step is in the sequence after she feels the hunger. I don't know. Suzanne tells me that she has known patients who have lived for years on nutritional drinks. But I can't imagine this is a good thing."

Tina sighs. I know she hears the worry in my voice. "Well, you hang in there, honey. She'll have a good meal today. Get some real protein into her. And tell your mom Happy Mother's Day from me, okay?"

"Do you remember Tina?" I ask my mother. "Remember, my friend who works for the airlines?"

I can almost see my mother searching her uncooperative database to locate Tina. When she does, she smiles. "Oh, she's such a lovely girl. How is she?"

"She's having a baby," I tell my mother.

"Is she married?" my mother asks.

"Yes, for a couple of years now, Mom."

"Well, that's good. She's such a lovely girl. What was her name again?"

"Tina.

"Yes. I like her."

"Tina asked me to wish you Happy Mother's Day."

"Where does she live?"

"New Hampshire."

"Too bad she is so far away."

"That's for sure."

"What did you tell me she did, again?"

"She is a flight attendant. And she's having a baby."

"Oh—is she married?"

"Yes, Mom—"

"She's such a lovely girl. But I wouldn't want a scandal!" My mother laughs. "When is the baby due?" she asks me.

"December."

"December," she repeats. "What month is it now?"

"May."

"May."

I am pretty certain that my mother has lost track of the conversation. "How about lunch?" I ask her. "Where do you want to go?"

"Honey, my hip really hurts today. I was thinking maybe we could stay here."

"You don't want to go out to eat?" I'm blindsided by my mother's desire to stay put. Always, always, she wants to leave Sunrise. *Escape, get out of this damn place, eat some real food.*

"I just don't feel up to it. Do you mind if we stay in, Katie?"

∽

We stay in. We eat Mother's Day dinner in the kitchen of the Aspen cottage. It is an improvement over our ill-fated Christmas dinner, and perhaps because I am seated at the table with her, my mother eats her meal. Or at least she nibbles on a little of everything. I am the token daughter in the room on this

Mother's Day. Many, but not most, of the residents are out with families on this special Sunday. But more than I would have expected are here, eating lamb chops. My mother's friend Geri sits across from us, chatting up a storm.

"She's a busybody." That was my mother's first impression of Geri, who zoomed around in a motorized wheelchair and wasn't shy about stating her opinions about everything and everybody. When my mother discovered that Geri was a retired teacher, she softened. They began to share their stories and spend more time together. My mother, always gifted at gathering information, found a repository in Geri, whose memory remained more or less intact. If my mother told her something, Geri would remember it for her—and happily spread the news.

After lunch, Geri invites us back to her room. I sit on the edge of the bed while my mother settles into the single armchair. I compliment Geri on her decor—heavy on crocheted items, but homey. "I've been thinking about painting the walls," she says. "I love your mother's pink room."

"I'm the only one in the place with a pink room," my mother declares.

"Everyone loves it," Geri tells me. "What color do you think would look good in here?"

After some discussion of how Geri might spiff up her room, my mother is ready to go. She stands, takes a single step, and begins to fall. Not thinking, only doing, I am on my feet. Gravity pushes us down, but I am in control of the descent. My mother is lowered to the ground, my arms wrapped around her rib cage, supporting her under the armpits.

"Pull the emergency cord." Geri obeys while I stay on the floor with my mother. I was able to support her weight going down, but I know I can't get her off the floor on my own. And I'm worried about how that fall happened. I've already scheduled an appointment for the coming week for my mother to be evaluated for a walker. I've got my mother on board by showing her the cart-style walkers that are much cooler than your standard-issue aluminum models. They boast built-in seats and front-hanging baskets to haul your stuff.

"That might prove convenient," my mother had agreed, repeating her formal turn of phrase with every recycle of our conversation. I only hope she can learn—and remember—to use the brakes.

"How do you feel?" I ask my mother now.

"A little sick to my stomach," she answers.

"How's your hip?"

"Fine," she says, sounding surprised. "You caught me."

"I did."

∽

A few minutes later, help arrives, and then a wheelchair. We get my mother up and into the chair, wheel her down the hall to her room. She is able to move from the chair to the bed on her own. The nurse on duty checks her vital signs, takes her blood pressure—acceptable. She suggests Tylenol in case my mother begins to feel achy, and I suggest ginger ale for her nausea. An aide produces both, and my mother, propped up in her bed, insists she'll be fine. "But I feel sick to my stomach," she adds.

"Do you remember what happened before you fell? Did you feel weak?" I ask her.

"I guess my hip just went out." There is a note of uncertainty in my mother's reply that I recognize: she's forgotten the fall.

"But your hip doesn't hurt now?" the nurse asks.

"No, I just feel a bit nauseous."

"Stay still," the nurse advises. "We're going to come in and check on you every hour tonight, okay, Anne?"

I sit with my mother. "Drink the ginger ale, Mom," I remind her every few minutes. She takes a sip.

"Uummm, that tastes good," she says with every swallow, but never, without prompting, does she take another sip.

Two or three Boosts a day—is anyone making certain she drinks the whole bottle? She may need more reminders to eat and drink. I suspect she may have fallen not because her hip gave out or because she tripped on the rug, but because she was too weak to walk.

"Do you feel like an ice cream?" I ask my mother about an hour after the fall. I know there are Hoodsies in the kitchen freezer.

"I'd love one."

After ice cream, some water, another visit from the nurse, and some more ginger ale, I say goodbye to my mother. I reassure her that we'll get her hip checked out, that we'll have her walking soon enough, maybe with one of those cool red carts we saw. I remind her to pull the cord if she needs to use the bathroom, because just for tonight, the staff wants her to use the wheelchair. "Do you want to pee now, before I go?"

"Kathleen!" she says. "I raised you better than that."

"Pardon me. Would you like to me to say 'urinate'? Is that better?"

"Thank you, but I do not have to use the john," she says in her mock-snotty voice. I take her half-serious, half-joking propriety as a sign that she is feeling a little better.

"You're sure?"

"Yes, dear," she says. "I'm fine."

♈

Two days later, I get another early morning call from the nurse at Sunrise. After she fills me in, I ask her to put my mother on the phone. "Mom, your blood pressure is way up again. I've asked for an ambulance to take you to the hospital. You'll get there before I do, but this way you'll get right into the emergency room. I'm going to get in my car right now and meet you there. Okay?"

"You'll be there?"

"You'll get there first, but I'll be there, Mom. I have to drive up from the Cape. Mom, I know the ambulance is scary, but we'll get better service this way."

"I feel lousy, Katie."

"I know, Mom. That's why we're going to send you to the hospital in an ambulance, okay? You'll get right in and I'll meet you there." I stay on the phone, recycling with her, hoping that the one thing that will stay with her is that I will be there soon. When the EMTs arrive, we say good-bye. "I'll see you at the hospital," I say one more time, feeling sick in my heart as I think of her, alone in the ambulance, alone in the ER.

∽

This time there is no question that my mother will be admitted, though we spend the better part of the day waiting for a bed. Finally she moves upstairs, onto a new floor of single rooms. There is an armchair and a little couch for visitors in her room, which has a beautiful view of piney woods. "If you have to be in the hospital for a few days," I say to my mother, "these are pretty nice digs."

She smiles weakly. Everything about my mother is weak right now. She hasn't been able to walk on her own since the fall—not because anything hurts, but because she feels unsteady whenever she tries to get on her feet. In two days' time—or for all I know, in the time it took to get to the hospital in the ambulance—her dementia seems to have kicked up several notches. She's confused, not entirely sure where she is or why. I think about what Suzanne has told me: stress and trauma can make a patient's Alzheimer's appear to be more advanced. That change isn't always permanent. I cling to that hope, watching my mother struggle to remember words.

"This is not who she is," I tell the first doctor, and the next and the next. "Yes, she has Alzheimer's, but she isn't this advanced. She doesn't suffer from disorientation or have trouble forming words. Please don't accept this as normal. Something else is happening here."

***

Days pass. My mother is hooked up to one IV delivering fluids, another delivering the various blood pressure meds the doctors seem to adjust and change at least once a day. Meanwhile, I wonder why my mother is unable to hold a cup or lift it to her lips. I visit her daily. Suzanne comes once with me and once on her own.

"I'm worried they are dismissing her. They think the Alzheimer's is so advanced. I tried to explain that she could dip into a deeper stage, told them what they see is either a result of stress or of something else going on. But one doctor told me Alzheimer's is unpredictable—his word—and that she's probably just further along than I realized."

"He's wrong. Alzheimer's follows a predictable path. That's one thing that distinguishes the disease from other forms of dementia. The lost awareness we see now is too dramatic. It's stress-induced," Suzanne says. She's visiting my mother at the hospital for the third time, this time arranging her visit to co-incide with mine. She considers the situation with the doctor. "Maybe he'll listen to Stephanie." Stephanie, a.k.a. Dr. Lim-bert, has been checking in with me and with the doctors on my mother's case, but her capacity to influence the situation is limited without admitting privileges at this hospital.

More tests, more phone calls. After conferring with Su-zanne and Stephanie, I persuade the new doctor on my mother's case to test for a urinary tract infection. They are common in dementia patients, who forget their symptoms and therefore don't report them. They are also potentially life-threatening when left untreated. "It didn't show up on the urine sample we took when she was admitted," the doctor, a woman—and the most sympathetic of those I have encountered thus far—says to me, "but if you want me to retest, I will."

The retest shows a raging infection. They begin IV antibi-otics. At last we see some improvement. My mother's awareness returns. She starts joking again. By the time Jack visits, she is pleased to see him and happy with the selection of books he brings her—a volume of poetry and an old history book that belonged to their father. But she still can't lift a cup to her lips or even imagine getting out of bed to walk. The doctor orders physical therapy. "You know your mother has a lot of health is-sues," she says the next time we speak, "but I'm happy with her blood pressure, and she's really bounced back since she's been on the antibiotics. Let's see if the physical therapy helps her get back some of her mobility. We'll start here at the hospital, but you need to start looking into rehab facilities. Her insur-ance won't allow her to stay here much longer. I'll ask the social worker to go over a discharge plan with you."

The mention of a rehab facility isn't a surprise. My mother must be ambulatory before she can move back to Sunrise. She can use a walker or a wheelchair, but she has to be able to travel the halls without assistance. I've already talked to Stephanie to see if she has any recommendations. She sees patients regularly at three facilities. She recommends one for my mother. It's called Crystal Lake, and it is about fifteen minutes further from my house. A small price to pay for Dr. Limbert's continuing care.

"Our goal at Crystal Lake," Stephanie says, "will be to get your mother in shape for assisted living again. But this episode has taken its toll. We'll have to take it one day at a time."

One day at a time, Medicare allows us twenty-one days. After that, Crystal Lake—a skilled nursing facility with rehabilitation services—will run us almost four times the price of Sunrise. And the rent at Sunrise still comes due, whether my mother is hospitalized or in rehab—so long as we want to hold on to her space there. I weigh the financial implications in the light of the limited money we have to support my mother's ongoing living situation. It will be difficult for my mother to learn how operate a wheelchair or a walker. She's forgotten sequencing that she's known all her life, and any assistive device will require my mother to learn and remember a series of brand-new steps. On the other hand, she's shown dramatic improvement in the past several days. Maybe Suzanne can help me find a way to make sure my mother gets the fluids she needs every day.

When the rent comes due at Sunrise, I send the check. Giving up that bright pink room feels too much like giving up on my mother.

Chapter Twenty-one

Till It's Gone

"How do I get out of this place?"

It's a beautiful day in late May. My mother is seated in a wheelchair parked next to my bench. Mom likes the grounds at Crystal Lake. There is indeed a lake, though we can't see it from here, and there is a feeling of spaciousness—in part because there are three components to the campus: independent senior living, assisted living, and a rehabilitation and skilled nursing facility—in plainer words, a nursing home. That's where my mother is staying. I can't blame her for wanting out. In fact, I want her out—and more: I want her to want out.

"Drink your fluids," I instruct my mother. "Every chance you get, drink something. Drink this for starters," I say, pointing to the Dixie cup in her hand. She can hold a cup again and get it to her lips now, but she still doesn't remember to drink. "You got dehydrated, and that's why you felt so bad. You can't afford to let that happen again."

"What else?" she asks.

"Do your physical therapy. We need to get you moving—maybe with a walker, or even in a wheelchair, but you have to be ambulatory to get out of here."

"Okay. When do I start?"

"Tomorrow," I tell her, feeling hope in my heart even as I wheel her back into the nursing care I know she needs right now. "Drink your water," I remind her again.

Obedient, she takes another bird-sip. "This is delicious water."

✍

"She likes the cold water from the water cooler," I tell the nurse at the station on my way out. "And she likes Boost—I put a case of chocolate in the fridge—and she likes milk shakes and she likes ginger ale." My mother's tendency to forget to drink was noted in her file, and I want to arm the staff with information to keep her hydrated. Their method thus far—leaving a container the size of a large to-go cup filled with ice water on her bed tray with instructions to drink it—is not yielding great results. She isn't dehydrated yet, but she isn't drinking the water either.

The nurses I've met at Crystal Lake are pleasant and willing to listen. But they are overworked, hurried much of the time. When they aren't administering medication off the rolling med cart, they are occupied with piles of paperwork. My sense is that I'll have to persuade their juniors—the certified nursing assistants—to take an interest in reminding my mother to drink her fluids.

In the three days since my mother has arrived at Crystal Lake, I've moved past suppressing my full-fledged horror to a state of still-horrified acceptance of her new surroundings. When the discharge manager at the hospital called me to say my mother was leaving, I hopped in my car and headed north, arriving about twenty minutes after my mother. It was evening—last-minute administrative complications had delayed her transfer. I followed the directions to my mother's room. I heard the murmur of television sets as I walked down the hall and tried not to look past the open doors into the other rooms.

My mother's first words: "Get me out of this place!"

I had been worried the change of scene might trigger another crisis of awareness. No, she was fully present. She could smell the smells and hear the man down the hall yelling, "Nurse! Nurse! I need help! Nurse! Nurse!"

"I brought you some clothes," I said.

"I don't need clothes! I need to get out of here."

"You won't be here long—a few weeks, tops. But you have to be mobile again before you can return to Sunrise."

"How long?"

"As soon as you can walk with a walker or operate a wheelchair, you can go back to your pink room."

My mother seemed to take this in. Then, tipping her head in the direction of the window, my mother whispered, "What the hell's up with her?" The far side of the room was packed with stuffed animals and dolls. Under a pile of crocheted afghans, a tiny woman was propped up on the pillows. My mother's roommate, I would later confirm, was in an advanced stage of Alzheimer's. She paid no attention to the deafening TV, but held tight to a baby doll and stared at nothing in particular. "She's loony," my mother declared, answering her own question.

The admissions director promised us a new room and a new roommate as soon as another bed freed up. In the meantime, the staff took to parking my mother in the open area by the nursing station for long stretches during the day. When I stepped off the elevator to see my mother, seated alone and listing to the left in her chair, I would swallow back the feelings of hopelessness that washed over me.

"It's freezing here."

"Let's go outside."

The early reports from the physical therapist were not optimistic. It seemed unlikely my mother would graduate to a walker. As I wheeled her onto the elevator, I thought, *We'll figure this out.* A folding wheelchair will fit into my hatch. I'll learn how to transfer her in and out of the car. We'll be able, soon, to go out to dinner. I'll get one of those tags for my car, and we'll be able to park in the handicapped spot when we go shopping. I imagined a future for us.

"Do you want to check out the apartments here? There's an open house."

"Why not?" my mother said.

I told the marketing rep that I hoped my aunt might come to live with my mother after she was out of rehab. It wasn't exactly a lie, just an expression of hopefulness ungrounded in any reality. She showed us a roomy two-bedroom. We thanked her and took the literature.

"I could never afford that place," my mother said when we were outside again.

"Probably not," I agreed. "But maybe someplace smaller. Should we check out the assisted living? I'm pretty sure the lake is behind that building."

"I'd love to see the lake," my mother agreed.

We were greeted in the lobby.

"We were thinking my mom might want to live here after she completes her rehab," I told the community representative. I was thinking I might be able to spring her from the nursing facility sooner if she were moving just across the parking lot. I was thinking it was possible that my mother might prefer the setting. I was thinking that I really wanted my mother to see the elusive Crystal Lake.

"Go ahead and have a look around," the woman suggested. "I'll give you some literature when you're on your way out. And we can make an appointment for a formal tour if you're inter-ested in seeing some of the rooms."

I wheeled my mother toward a large parlor where several women were sitting. I introduced my mother, and each of the ladies introduced themselves, welcoming us into their circle. "Oh, you'll get the best therapy over there," one woman reas-sured my mother. "They do an excellent job." The other women nodded their agreement. Stories were told of rehabilitation and release, stories that made us both feel better.

"I hope you can join us here soon," one of the women said as we excused ourselves to go outdoors.

Down in a patio area, we found another group of women, just as friendly and outgoing. "It's down there, past the trees," a tiny lady with a bright floral top told me when I asked about the lake. "There's a path. But we like to sit up here." We chatted with the outdoor ladies until my mother began to feel a chill.

We never made it to the lake, but it was almost enough to know we were close.

Chapter Twenty-two

DNR

How is it, I wonder—not for the first time—that we adapt so readily to changing circumstances? Our parents move from youth to age, and age becomes the norm. Who were those slim, vibrant, smiling people in the honeymoon pictures? They were younger than we are—younger, it sometimes feels, than we ever were. Who were they? And who were we?

No matter. We brush our hair out of our eyes, the cobwebby half-memories out of our minds. We soldier on. Our elders move from strength to debility, and debility becomes the norm. We accept their decline, we call on our own strength, we cease to question who they were and focus instead on who they are—now. We see their need. And we answer it.

My mother, two months ago, was not strong or healthy. But she was not in a wheelchair. Two weeks ago she was in a wheelchair, but itching to get out of it and out of this place. Today my mother is asleep in a bed by the window of her new room at Crystal Lake. She has pulled her knees up toward her chest, and I adjust the comforter I have brought from her room at Sunrise. I've decorated her new digs with photographs and get-well cards. On the bedside table and the bureau, I have installed two of her favorite lamps.

Harry helped me move my mother's stuff out of Sunrise,

where her friends asked for her and wished her well. "She won't be able to move back for some time," I told them, "and we just can't afford to hold on to the room." They accepted this; her friend Geri also accepted a small table and my mother's mini-fridge. She gave me a cane that she'd covered in patriotic fabric as a gift for my mother. I thanked Geri, hugged her, and knew my mother would never use that cane. Nor would she return to her pink room.

My mother is dying. It could be weeks, but not months. She was released to rehab, but she will not be rehabilitated. As I watch her, fitful in her half-sleep, I am adapting, yet again, to this new reality. As much as I want her to sit up in bed and ask for a Boost, I understand that three Boosts a day will not save my mother's life. Her kidneys have shut down. Her other organs will soon follow. And there will be no medical interventions on her behalf. In my capacity as my mother's health care proxy, I've signed a Do Not Hospitalize order and a Do Not Resuscitate order—the third one this year.

When the admissions coordinator at Crystal Lake brought me the paperwork, I signed it without hesitation. Once again, I seem to have adapted to a new normal: my mother is dying, and I will not stand in her way.

I remember that when my mother was in Sunrise, I delayed signing that first DNR. "You wouldn't be doing your mother any favors to allow resuscitation in the event of cardiac arrest," Dr. Limbert had told me after the tumors were located on my mother's left lung. I knew she was right, but I was bothered by the fact that the DNR would be posted on the back of my mother's door at Sunrise.

"The paperwork on the door allows the EMTs to know right away whether or not they should begin CPR," the wellness coordinator explained to me.

"I understand the . . . efficiency . . . of having the order on the back of the door—but I worry that my mother will find it disturbing."

"Many of the residents have the order in place. It doesn't seem to bother anybody."

My mother, I thought, is not anybody. For one thing, she could still read. She would forget what she read, but that DNR, I imagined, would catch her eye every time she stepped out of her room. She would see my signature on a form that said Don't Save My Mother's Life. "How would you feel seeing a written reminder of your mortality every time you left your office?" I asked.

Silence. The wellness coordinator had decided to treat that as a rhetorical question. I forged ahead. "Could we put it in a manila envelope, at least?"

"Well, the point is to make it clear right away to the fire department. That's why we leave it in plain sight. But I can look into this."

Within a week or two, the document was signed, placed in a manila envelope, and hung on the back of my mother's door— where my mother left it, never opening the envelope or seeming to wonder about its appearance.

A hospice-trained nurse named Mary—my grandmother's name—checks in, adjusts the pillow, pats my mother's hand, and talks to me. Mary is kind, compassionate, and seemingly heaven-sent. She is determined to keep my mother comfortable. *Safe and comfortable*, I think to myself. It's been my mantra these last few years. And now, I realize, the safest, most comfortable place my mother can be—is far, far away from here.

ᔄ

My cell phone rings early the next morning. I'm at Tina's house in New Hampshire. I drove up yesterday afternoon, stopping to visit my mother on the way. I have a bookstore client in a nearby town, and I've postponed twice already. I will see him today, drive back this evening, stop on my way home to see my mother again. I recognize the number on the caller ID. Crystal Lake. It's Mary.

"I wanted to let you know, Kate, that your mother's condition changed overnight. I came in around four thirty this morning—earlier than I usually do, but I was called in. Your mom seemed to be in pain, and the fentanyl patch didn't seem to be taking care of it anymore."

Doctor Limbert had prescribed the patch a few days earlier. "It's hard to know for sure the source of your mother's pain," she had said to me, "but based on the way Anne is acting, I believe it is severe. Unless you have objections, I will treat the pain with opioids. We'll start with a patch containing fentanyl, but we will always have the option for an oral dose of morphine or even a drip."

The patch seemed to have a beneficial effect. For a couple of days my mother seemed more relaxed. She was too weak to do much talking, but she remained engaged for short visits.

"So I put in a call to Dr. Limbert," Mary continues. "She came in around six and agreed with me that your mom was in more pain, and so she prescribed some morphine by mouth, and we gave her a dose. She seemed a lot more comfortable after that. Dr. Limbert said she could have it as often as every hour, if that was okay with you. She asked me to call for your okay." In the pause before I answer, Mary adds, "So far she hasn't needed much, just a little, but we just want her to stay comfortable. We don't want her in any pain."

"Yes." I hear myself repeating the words one more time.

"I want her, most of all, to be comfortable, and safe. Before we hang up, I tell Mary I'm working in New Hampshire today. "I will stop to see my mother on my way back to the Cape this evening. Please let her know that I'm coming, will you?"

⌁

All lampshades—whether cloth or, God forbid, paper—are ugly, according to my mother, and must be avoided at all costs. Ditto for overhead lighting, doubly offending the eye—ugliness paired with exuberant brightness. In her decorating heyday, my mother acquired seventeen lampshade-free Fenton glass table lamps. In her collection are ruby red, satin pink, milky green, buttery yellow. Some are missing the upper section, and she has at least one upper globe without a matching bottom; but for the most part, these glass and brass lapses in her good taste have survived many moves intact. Her brother Jack thinks they are hideous. I can imagine one or two in the right setting: an old Victorian B and B. But seventeen? Yes, seventeen. In my mother's four-room Cape Cod cottage.

Without a trace of guilt, I sold two at the "estate" sale. Two more—the ruby red Bordello models—are with my friend Tony, who promises to sell them for me on eBay. Eleven are packed in bubble wrap and stored in my basement. That leaves two— matching pink satin glass, in large and small. They are glowing now, soft, serene. It's close to nine o'clock, and the overhead lights have been turned off. My mother is awake and bathed in pale pink light. As I bend over to give her a kiss, I am a convert. The lamps are beautiful, the lighting perfect. Perhaps, I think, I'll take one out of the basement and move it into my living room.

My mother holds my hand. "Katie," she says.

"I'm here, Mom. Can I get you anything? Some Boost? Some ginger ale?"

"Ow. Oww."

"Are you in pain? Should I call the nurse?"

"Ow, Katie."

"Okay, just give me one minute. Let me see about some pain medication, Mom. I'll be right back."

The nurse checks her chart. "Your mother hasn't asked for anything in a few hours," she tells me. "She can definitely have another dose. Let me get it, and I'll be right down there."

I return to my mother's room, hold her hand, rub her shoulder, tell her the medicine is coming. All she says is, "Ow."

"It will be okay, Mom. The nurse will be here in a minute."

When she arrives, the nurse switches on the overhead lights. She gives my mother a few drops of morphine. "This will help," she tells her, patting her other hand.

"Ow," my mother says, but with less intensity. In the bright light, my mother looks gray, but I can see that she is beginning to relax.

"Dr. Limbert says she can have the morphine every hour, but she really hasn't needed much for the pain," the nurse says.

"Well, she may need more now," I say. "She was clearly in a lot of pain when I arrived. Can you make a point to check her every hour overnight?"

"We will," she promises. "Shall I turn out the lights?"

"Please," I say, turning back to my mother. She seems tiny. I call her "Big Mom" whenever I am speaking to Bix. The first time she heard the term, my mother was insulted. "That makes me sound like a large lady."

"You could never be confused with a large lady," I reassured her at the time. Now I wish she were large—or at least that she had been larger when she began this journey. I wish that she had more reserves, more resiliency. My skinny-mini mother is wasting away. It seems possible that she might just disappear. But it isn't that easy to leave these physical bodies. We cling to life, limited though it may be. We fight. For what? To live to drink another Boost?

It's time, I realize, and I need to let my mother know. I need to tell her I'll be okay, that she need not hang around on my account. Because I suspect that despite her pain, her advancing dementia, she still worries about me. Even when we haven't always gotten along, we have faced the world together. Now I understand that we are connected—always have been, always will be. No one else in the world will be my mother.

I'm not sure she will hear me, or if she hears me, that she will register what I am saying.

"Mom," I say. "I love you. And I'm going to be fine. Please don't worry about me." I pause, collecting myself.

Weeping these words won't do. I must sound convincing.

"I'll be just fine. But you—you're tired, and you're in pain. And you don't have to be. You can go to a place where there is no pain. No confusion. Just let go, Mom. Go there."

I turn my head away, blow my nose.

"Mom," I say, stroking her back. "I love you," I repeat. "I want you to get some rest. Just relax. Please don't worry about leaving me. I promise I'll be okay."

My mother is quiet. I pull her covers up under her chin, turn off one of the lamps. "Goodnight, Mom," I whisper, leaning over to give her a kiss goodbye.

Chapter Twenty-three

Irish Wake

When you throw a wake, you don't control the guest list. You make a million small decisions about how the deceased will be presented and honored. You select a casket, pick out prayer cards, specify a charity for memorial donations, make photo collages of your loved one's life, and tell the florist you will accept no lilies. You set the date, time, and place and do your best to get the word out to the folks you know. You run an obituary in several papers, hoping to inform the people you don't know personally or don't know how to contact.

You get your hair done, because you know your mother would be appalled if you didn't. You decide what to wear: a short, black pencil skirt; a silk chiffon blouse with a swirly print of black, gold, and teal and a rosette on the collar; sheer black tights; black nubuck pumps. The combination is unconventional, but still tasteful. You want something that doesn't look like death. You want something you could wear to a cocktail party. "Oh, Katie—*très chic.*" That's what you want your mother to say, in that mock-dramatic voice she uses when she says a few words in another language.

The thing is, you don't invite anyone to attend a memorial event. You may expect family members and some close friends, but beyond that circle of predictability lies a whole universe of people who may or may not hear the news, may or may not show up. You might know their names. You might not. You might be pleased to see them, to meet them at last. Or—as is the case when Mr. Russell Nibs introduces himself to me—you may be horrified and astonished, even as you smile and shake his hand.

Mom, I have no idea why he's here! I swear!

In my *Romper Room* theology, I'm unclear about whether my deceased mother is listening. Eventually, I'm pretty sure, she will be able to, in some sense, hear me. But right now? I'm guessing she's going through an extensive adjustment period. Still, I apologize, because Mr. Russell Nibs—tall and hale and well into his seventies—is also the boy who scattered tacks on my mother's piano bench. It was an end-of-the-year student recital, and he was her page turner and her tormentor. My mother, trained to always act the lady, seated herself and played her piece. Pricked by tacks, consumed by nerves, my mother bade farewell to musical performance. She never played again.

I've heard the story of Russell Nibs and the tacks on the piano bench on many occasions, though I think I would remember it even if I'd heard it just once. I understand the debilitating potential of preperformance anxiety. I wouldn't want to deal with tacks on my seat as well. Besides, the name is unforgettable. Russell Nibs. Here he is, in the flesh—sixty-something years after his irrevocable act.

He speaks before I can offer up a conflicted *thank you for coming.*

"I'm a friend of your uncle Jack's."

Just like that. I bet he doesn't remember the piano bench incident at all. It was just one small prank among many, a joke on the sister of his friend Jack. It has occurred to me in the past to wonder whether Russell Nibs had a crush on my mother, if the tacks on the bench were the piano recital equivalent of dipping her pigtails in his inkwell. Now I think not. He's a friend of my uncle Jack's.

Mom, I intone silently, *I'm sorry about this one.*

Here to balance the influence of the once-youthful prankster is another guest: the superintendent of schools for a good deal of my mother's career. I've never met him, but he was the central character—and often the hero—of many stories I heard my mother tell. He encouraged my mother's educational crusades and supported her time and time again before the school committee. "Your mother was a firecracker," he says to me, right after saying how sorry he is.

"She was, wasn't she?" I say. "Thank you so much for coming."

                                      ⁀

Fionah was with me when the phone call came. It was just before three on Thursday afternoon. A few minutes later and we would have missed the call. We were about to leave for Crystal Lake.

"I've got the harp in the car, and I promised I'd play for your mother."

Fionah had met my mother only a couple of times, but had taken to her right away. "She's a brilliant woman, now, isn't she? It's so apparent, even with her illness." I was grateful for Fionah's assessment of my mother's intelligence. She seemed to see through all the foggy present and right into my mother's essence. Perhaps that was why she offered to play—nothing formal, just a salon concert for my mother and her friends. But Mom was hospitalized before we worked it out.

That Thursday afternoon—with my mother hovering between life and death—I worried that solo harp might sound too much like Heaven. "Maybe I'll take my flute, too," I suggested to Fionah. "We can play some duets."

"Grand," she said. She followed me into my bedroom, settling into the rocker as I gathered up the flute, some music, a folding stand. And then my office phone rang. It stopped shy of four rings, and I didn't get there in time. I checked the caller ID: Crystal Lake. I was about to begin dialing back when my personal line rang.

"Kate, it's Mary."

"She's gone." The words were out before I could stop them. Not even a question. I just knew.

"Yes, I'm so sorry. Just a few minutes ago."

"We were just leaving to come see her—"

"I'm sorry, Honey. But she had a good day. We got her dressed this morning, in the outfit her sister sent. And Dr. Limbert came in and visited with her for a while. I think they had a nice talk. I've been checking on her all day. We didn't expect this so soon, but I guess she was ready. She was peaceful, Kate. It wasn't hard for her."

"Oh. Okay." I say, just to fill the silence.

"Do you know what you want us to do?"

Do? It took me a moment to understand what she was asking. "Oh. Yes. Yes, please. We're using Cartmell's in Plymouth. What should I do now?"

"Nothing right away, Kate. We'll call the funeral home, and they'll get back in touch with you. I'll personally take care of your mother's things. You can pick them up any time that's convenient. I'm working all day tomorrow." She paused, as if she knew I was having trouble taking in all the information. "Kate, I'm so sorry for your loss. Your mother was a lovely lady."

After the call, there were more calls. I called my mother's siblings, Jack and Rose. "You're kidding!" Rosemary said when

I told her the news. I remembered saying the same two words to my stepbrother John when he called me twenty-four years before to tell me my father had died. We say inane things when we are confronted with bad news. And death, I've learned, is always unexpected. Even when you know it's coming.

If only we were kidding. If only it were some big, giant, cosmic joke.

Before I could notify anyone else, someone from the funeral home called. "We already have you down for an appointment tomorrow afternoon," he said.

After visiting with my mother on Wednesday, Suzanne had suggested I begin to make arrangements. "It will be easier to make decisions in advance than it will in the thick of everything," she had said, offering to come along.

The next morning, after booking the appointment, I'd sat down to write my mother's obituary. "I imagine you'll want to write it yourself." Suzanne had said. She was right; I could trust no one to sum up my mother's life in three hundred words or less.

When the phone call from Mary came that morning, I wondered whether my actions had sent entirely the wrong signal to the universe. I had wanted to be ready, yes. But, no I was not prepared. We never are.

"If you can make it in the morning instead," the funeral director said, we can hold the viewing on Sunday and the funeral on Monday."

"Yes. It will be easier for folks to get here on the weekend," I heard myself say.

By Friday morning, Fionah and Suzanne and Cindy and Tina had formed a circle of protection around me. Cindy, from her home in New Jersey, made calls to a list of friends and colleagues—my mother's and mine. Suzanne drove me to the funeral home, helping me make a multitude of inane decisions. Tina made her way from New Hampshire to Cape Cod to stay with me through Sunday. Fionah picked up my mother's things from the nursing home and accompanied me to the florist. From there, I called Cindy with the floral and funeral details so that she could send out specifics in a follow-up e-mail to the people she had already contacted.

For the past three days, I have occupied the passenger seat—first in Suzanne's car, then Fionah's, and this morning Tina's. I have had sleepover company in the guest room, where my mother's bed from Sunrise now resides. Food has appeared, though I have not prepared it. The rules of early mourning: do not drive; do not sleep in the house alone; do not cook.

Perhaps all the taking care of me is what allows me now to act the hostess at my mother's Irish wake. I welcome each visitor, introduce people to each other. We have three rooms, and in each room is an easel with a collage. Tina and I made them yesterday, taping memorabilia to the poster board: my mother's fifth-grade report card, all A's; a program from a play she directed; her college portrait; a black-and-white photo of my mother, sleeveless and in Bermuda shorts, holding me.

"What a beauty she was!" I hear variations on this expression again and again. I remember a moment a few years ago when Tony came across my mother's college graduation photograph. "Your mother was a babe!" he said. My mother *was* a babe. The sun and cigarettes drew lines on her face; the white strands lightened her wavy auburn hair, but my mother's big blue eyes sparkled, drew you in, and her laughter could fill a room. If she were here—and not just in body—my mother would be pleased at the turnout. She would not want us to be grim. She would not want hushed silence or reverence. She would want stories to be told. Stories that honor her strength and her beauty, stories she had forgotten about herself. "I did that?" she would have asked us, again and again. And again and again I would have assured her, *Yes, Mom, you did.*

∽

The Kate Care Committee works in relays. Suzanne to Fionah to Tina to Shannon back to Fionah to Cindy, who meets me Monday morning at the funeral home. I feel less like a hostess today, and I am surprised by the visitors who come by before the funeral. Two of my mother's college classmates show up, and so does her longtime secretary. The family trickles in. Theresa wraps me in a big hug, and I silently thank my father for marrying this generous spirit. Her son, my stepbrother John, has agreed to be a pallbearer. My mother's coffin will be borne by a blended party of six: John, my stepsister Vicki, my cousins Julie, Justin, and Joshua, and my friend Harry.

While she was at Sunrise, my mother and the Catholic Church came to terms, perhaps thanks to her process of forgetting. She began attending Mass again. On Friday, the funeral director asked me what type of funeral I wanted. "Catholic," I said, feeling certain that my mother would want a Mass. Strangely, so do I. I want the big church, the robed priest, the incense, the beauty and rightness of the ritual.

I have not hired a limo for the short drive to the church. Instead I will ride with Cindy. We are at the head of the line, waiting in the driveway for the casket to be loaded into the hearse, when one of the funeral directors knocks on my window.

"The Celtic cross," she says. "She's wearing it. You'll want that, won't you?"

In truth, I'd thought to bury it with my mother. She wore it always. She bought it in Ireland—or not. In my hesitation, Cindy jumps in.

"Yes—you'll want to have it, Kate."

"I will?"

"Yes, I think you will. If you don't want to keep it, you can give it to Rosemary."

The funeral director says, "I do think you'll want to have it."

"Okay," I say. "Good."

∽

Do not stand at my grave and weep.
I am not there.

In a few minutes, after everyone is seated, Fionah will sing those words. I had selected the poem, written in the 1930s by Mary Elizabeth Frye, for my mother's prayer card, but I was unaware that several composers have set the words to music. "I promised I'd play for your mother," Fionah had reminded me. She helped me make the musical selections. Traditional and not. Harp, piano, two voices. No organ, please. I was emphatic on that point when I spoke to the music director. Just like no lilies. Death requires no more reminders.

After the pallbearers hoist the casket up the steps and into the church, the procession begins: two priests carrying incense; the casket, now on wheels but still attended by the pallbearers; finally, the family members. There is a pause in the proceedings when a vanload of Sunrise residents enters through the side door. I'm glad to see them. Now I feel like this beautiful church is filled with people who loved my mother at every stage of her life.

Yesterday at the wake, I welcomed an old friend of my mother's. "Our last conversation, I'm not sure she knew who I was," she told me. I was instantly angry. My mother would have recognized her longtime friend—had her friend bothered to keep up with her these past couple of years. I'd contacted her more than once, suggesting she visit my mother, take her out for an ice cream. I provided directions, instructions, helpful hints, reassured her that Sunrise is not a sad place, not a nursing home. I'd even offered to come along for moral support. I knew my mother would have been thrilled by a visit, would have enjoyed spending time with her friend again. But she never made contact. It just wasn't in her. I understood, on one level, that she missed the brilliant woman she knew, that she thought of her friend Anne as an almost separate person from the woman who repeated herself on the telephone. She wasn't the only person in my mother's circle with an inability to connect those dots. But she made the mistake of remarking on my mother's impaired memory at exactly the wrong moment.

"Oh, I am sure she recognized you," I said. "She might have forgotten your conversation a few minutes later, or repeated a story to you a couple of times, but she would have known you. She loved you."

Even as the words left my mouth, I felt bad about saying them. But I was unwilling to absolve her. My mother's friend had inadvertently awakened the lioness within. *My mother, even with an imperfect memory, was still deserving of attention, love, affection, and your respect.* That's what I was really saying.

Now, watching the Sunrise ladies get settled in the pews, I feel like the most important guests have arrived. The people who loved my mother, valued her presence, the people who would feel nostalgic not only for "the old Anne." They would miss the most recent version—the Anne they knew, the

Anne, they will tell me after the Mass, who made them laugh every day.

"Jack," I hear my aunt Jane whisper, "go up by Kate." But the procession restarts, and he can't get to me. Cindy tries too, but she ends up just behind me. At the head of the line, I walk alone. Behind my mother's casket. Walking slowly, staring at the polished maple box that holds what remains of my mother. It all becomes real to me. My mother is dead.

The tears come. Tears I will weep for days, weeks, months, years. Tears that I wipe off my cheek with the Kleenex that Cindy hands me. Tears I hide. I look down at the floor, count the tiles, the steps, until we reach the front pew.

> *Do not stand at my grave and weep.*
> *I am not there. I do not sleep.*
>
> *I am a thousand winds that blow.*
> *I am the diamond's glint of snow.*
> *I am the sunlight on ripened grain.*
> *I am the autumn's gentle rain.*
> *When you wake in the morning's hush,*
> *I am the uplifting rush*
> *Of quiet birds in circled flight*
> *I am the stars that shine at night.*
>
> *Do not stand at my grave and cry.*
> *I am not there. I did not die.*

Chapter Twenty-four

After Words

I dream of my mother. She doesn't speak to me in spirit or hand out sage advice. No, these are dreams filled with mundane activities—visits to eye doctors, hairdressers, dentists; shopping trips to CVS; the occasional dinner out. Activities designed to remind me, just before the dream ends, that my mother is dead. Often I speak the words aloud: "Oh, right, she's dead." My voice when I speak these words is calm, matter-of-fact, neutral. Never do I say *passed away* or *gone* or *in spirit* in reference to my mother's state. No euphemisms in these dreams. Sometimes the words are spoken by a voice I do not recognize. By an unaffected, uninflected voice, I am reminded one more time: my mother is dead.

As if I might forget.

My mother died on the summer solstice. A Thursday. Her funeral was the following Monday.

On the first Thursday, on the first Monday, I travel back in time seven days. On Thursday I remember writing her obituary. I remember the phone call. I remember she died. Without me there. On Monday I remember getting up that morning, showering, getting ready, trying to get a little food into my stomach. I remember walking behind my mother's coffin. I remember the music, beautiful and sad.

Which day is worse? Monday or Thursday? Thursday is worse, I think, until Monday comes around.

Two weeks ago today. Three weeks ago today. I wonder how long I'll think this way. I can't imagine that I will mark my mother's passing on every Thursday for the rest of my life. But on the other hand, I can imagine this will go on for some time.

The distance from death may be like the distance from birth in this way. We age infants first in days, then weeks, before we shift to measuring in months. Even after a child's first birthday, we still keep track in months: *fifteen months*; *nineteen months*. With that second birthday, we begin to calculate in years and sometimes half years. Does the math get too difficult? Or does the addition of a single month become less relevant?

I am in the phase of counting weeks. Two weeks. Two weeks ago today, in the morning, I wrote my mother's obituary. Two weeks ago, in the afternoon, my mother died.

"Oh right, she's dead," my dream self says.

No poetry in that.

∽

"How are you doing?" Cindy asks me.

"How are you doing?" Tina asks me.

There are times when I start crying and cannot stop. These episodes sneak up on me without warning. I find myself weeping those body-wracking sobs that echo in the house. Bix always comes to find me. Patting him, I calm myself. "I'm sorry I woke you from your nap," I say by way of apology.

Most of the time I am just sad. Sad and subdued. I find myself reflecting on the arc of my mother's life. Wishing I could rewrite it. Alter it. Wondering what small shift, what path not taken, might have changed the course of her living. And her dying. I question myself compulsively about the decisions I made on her behalf. Should I have treated the cancer? Pushed her to undergo dialysis? Should I have tried harder to find a place where we both could have lived?

If I'd known.

I travel the dead-end theoreticals.

"You did everything you could," Cindy tells me.

"You were a wonderful daughter," Tina tells me.

Mostly, I believe them. Even as I revisit my decisions, I know that I made them with an open heart, with good intentions, with my mother's best interests in mind. The sadness, as it settles, returns to the wish that my mother could have lived a better, easier, happier life.

∽

The dreams are changing. It seems a terrible mistake has been made. My mother is still alive. In these dreams there is no issue with her health, no reason why she would have to stay in the nursing home, no reason she couldn't return to Sunrise, except that I, in my misunderstanding of the situation, have moved her out, given up her room, spent the money we could have put toward her rent on a funeral. The dreams do not show me precisely how or why she might have been mistaken for dead, but they suggest bureaucratic mishaps, misdiagnoses, an overexcited read of a situation that, in fact, was not dire. Only once—in the most disturbing of the variations—do I realize she has been buried alive. No matter, she returns.

For weeks, I experience and re-experience this dream-world combination of horror, guilt, and frantic worry. I grow used to this nighttime ritual, and I stop trying to figure out why I have to repeat this dream again and again. That's when a new dream shows up. In this one my mother speaks to me for the first time since she died. She tells me that she has always worried about my finances and that she wants me to use the money she left behind to create some financial security for myself.

Waking, I am aware there was not much cash left after I paid all my mother's bills. I suspect my dream mother may be as confused about money as my real mother was. I remember she envisioned for me a minimum security with an overstated value.

"You're going to be a rich bitch," she had a habit of saying when I visited her at Sunrise.

"How so?"

"When I'm gone, you'll get all of these." She would gesture toward the bureau where her Hummels were displayed. "And you can sell them. Then you'll be a rich bitch." She would smile—at the rhyme and, I think, at her risqué language—and maybe because she was managing to mix kindness with a dash of hostility in her choice of words.

I would remind her that she had once told me not to sell anything but to give away her things to people who would love them.

"Nah. Sell them. They'll make you rich."

They are boxed up in the basement now, those Hummels, their fate uncertain. I am not yet rich.

✍

Tina, in her final trimester, is at last free from nausea. She is energetic, and she looks fabulous. She comes to visit on my birthday, bearing gifts. She's full of plans. "Thanksgiving," she says. "Jonathan is flying, and I don't know if I'll be able to drive."

"My God, of course you aren't driving here, if that's what you mean—you're due two weeks later. What if you go early? I'll come to you."

"I know my kitchen isn't ideal. But can we make a turkey? And your mashed potatoes? And—"

"We'll make everything," I tell her.

I find myself looking forward to the holiday. It will be the first Thanksgiving without my mother, but on the other hand, it will be the last Thanksgiving before Tina's daughter is born. Maybe I feel lighter because I am borne up by Tina's visit. Or maybe it is the dream I had the night before my birthday. In this one, my mother and I are talking. Just chitchat, nothing of any real substance. She's lively, healthy, and possessed of all her faculties. She looks good. But the whole time we're talking, I know she is dead.

Finally I screw up the courage to ask her.

"What's it like, Mom—being dead?"

"Oh," she says, "it can be confusing. There are so many things you have to learn." She pauses, then brightens.

"But you know what's great about it? I can fly."

∽

Elise is born on a snowy Monday in December. Jonathan calls me with the news, his voice brimming with something that sounds like awe. "Everybody's fine," he reassures me. "Tina says you should stay put—don't drive in this weather. And oh—she told me to be sure to tell you the baby has prominent eyebrows."

The baby, Tina is telling me, looks like her husband.

"That's so funny." I'm laughing through my tears, thrilled—and also profoundly relieved—that Elise has made her way safely into the world. The baby girl with the prominent eye-brows represents hope, continuity, and balance in the universe. It's a tall order for a tiny package.

A tiny package who will make her presence known, early and often. By day, Baby Elise is uninterested in sleeping. She thrills and gurgles in company, but by late afternoon—exhausted—she turns cranky and inconsolable. Tina and Jonathan try swaddling and bouncing, with inconsistent results.

Consulting books on the subject, Tina reads that some babies need noise—specifically a loud, buzzy noise—to calm them. According to one expert, the reverberation of a vacuum cleaner in this new, outer world reminds them of the swishy sounds they heard in the womb. Because their hearing is not fully developed and their eardrums are still sheathed, babies experience the roar as something more like a purr. Not so for us grownups. When I visit, Tina and I sit in the sun-filled family room, sipping tea. There is no small talk over the deafening vacuum cleaner. We are content without words, grateful for the sleeping Baby Elise.

◈

Elise will never be a crib baby. She will move past the white noise and into a musical swing. Then, past the motion and into her mother's arms. Or her father's. Or, on some precious occasions, mine. Midway in the terrible twos, Leesie will consider napping in her own toddler bed, in her own room, the walls decorated with forest sprites and fairies. By that time, my house will be furnished with a secondhand high chair, an array of thirdhand toys. My car will have a car seat I found on Craigslist. Fionah, running errands with me after a summer away, will ask, "Kate, did I miss something really big while I was gone?"

We will laugh, but something really big has happened. Leesie has joined the family.

In the tradition of families, Leesie will name me herself: *Bop.*

"Bop! Bop!" she will shout every time she sees me. At first we will think it is a musical request, but in time we will understand that Bop is my name. It will supersede *Auntie Kate*, the honorific bestowed by Tina, and it will speak to our musical connection, forged when infant Elise wasn't listening to the vacuum cleaner (or later, the vacuum cleaner CD). Before she talks, Leesie will hum. Together we will sing silly songs that require only non-sense syllables—like *bop*. By the time she has turned two, Leesie will discover the basket of wooden flutes next to the piano. For me, she will select a Tibetan flute decorated with silver studs. I will give her the soprano recorder. We will march down the hallway and into the kitchen, making joyful noise.

One summer night when Leesie is nearing three, I will ask, "Shall we take a postprandial stroll?"

"Okay," she will say.

"Have you ever encountered that word?" I ask Tina.

Tina, a reader and a thinker, has not. I'm not surprised. It's arcane, a bit archaic, and one of my mother's favorite words. She taught it to me when I was just a little girl. Never mind that her favorite usage was linked with the word *cigarette*. It means *after-dinner*, or more precisely, *after-meal*. As I unbuckle Leesie from her high chair, I will remember how my mother gifted me with words—big words—when I was just a little thing. And in the tradition of families, I will pass that gift along to Tina's daughter.

"Posprandal," Leesie will offer up.

"That's right. It means after we've had dinner. And you

know what *stroll* is—a walk." Leesie will nod, paying me close attention. "So I wondered if you wanted to take an after-dinner walk for—"

"Ice cream!" Leesie fills in the blank and waits for me to continue.

"You scream! We all scream for—"

"Ice cream!"

It's a warm night. But I'm also sure my mother is radiating her approval—of the vocabulary lesson and of my choice for dessert.

∽

When my mother died, I was forty-eight. Then forty-nine. Now I have achieved fifty years. Cindy, using her particular brand of magic and working from New Jersey, has secretly assembled close to thirty people in a Thai restaurant in Plymouth, Massachusetts, at six thirty on a Tuesday night. Jack and Jane are here, Harry and Tami, Fionah; Anne, taking photographs; my stepmom, Theresa, and my stepbrother, John; Tina, of course; and Elise, enchanted by the silver tiara with the glittering purple "50" on it. As I scan the well-wishers—friends, family, close colleagues—I realize: Cindy used the e-mail list I'd given her when my mother died. The folks she had notified of my mother's death, she has notified of this big anniversary of my birth. A poetic gesture, a way to transform sadness and death into life and celebration. I love her for it. But I still want to kill her for letting my secret out.

My mother always told me, "A lady never reveals her age."

A ridiculous and outmoded bit of advice. Or so I thought, until I turned—forty-ten.

But Cindy's list is not all-inclusive. Our band director, John, for example, was unaware of my changeover birthday when he programmed a piece for solo flute and band, *Autumn Soliloquy*, for our next concert. I've been a soloist once before with the band—about five years ago. John had consulted with me well in advance of my first featured performance. This time the music just appeared in my folder.

"That's you," he said, coming behind my stand and pointing to the words *Solo Flute*.

"Okay." I was thinking, *He won't make me play it tonight, at the first rehearsal of the season, sight-reading in front of the whole band.* But that's exactly what he did.

Nine weeks later, in my usual preconcert state of disarray, I do not feel older or wiser. But I remind myself as I stand and move into position: *You nailed this piece on the first read.*

John asks me with his eyes if I am ready, and I give a small nod, raising my flute to my lips. I inhale, long and deep. Then I play.

I play the slow, mournful passing of the summer season and the skittering of golden leaves. I play salt-air mist and November gray, the nostalgia we feel for the days gone by. I play time passing and the miraculous lightening of the sky that happens after an autumn rain. I play for my mother, for the sadness and beauty of her life, for everything she gave me, including—because she thought it was prettier than a clarinet—a shiny silver flute.

Acknowledgments

Suzanne Faith suggested I write about my experience with my mother, and Jay Leutze assured me—early and often—that I could. Julia Lord believed in the music and in me, in the writing and in the work. Bob Wyatt first spoke the words—*remembered music*—that grew into the title. Tom Hallock persuaded Helene Atwan to have a look, thereby connecting me to the best editor a book—or a writer—could ask for. At Beacon Press, the book received expert care in the hands of Bob Kosturko, P.J. Tierney, Susan Lumenello, Kathy Carter, Pam MacColl, Caitlin Meyer, Alyssa Hassan, and Crystal Paul. These gracious early readers were willing to share their enthusiasm: Chuck Robinson, Keebe Fitch, Brian Woodbury, Gayle Shanks, and Barbara Mead.

Many friends, mom-care partners, family members, and musical colleagues appear in these pages, and many good souls remain behind the narrative curtain. My thanks are with everyone who is present in my life.